FROM MISERY TO HOPE

BY

ROBERT D. PALMER AND **KARY YOUMAN**

From Misery To Hope
by
Robert D. Palmer and Kary Youman

Editing/Formatting: Gloria Palmer *(movinonup57@yahoo.com)*

Published by: Tenth House Publishing
                  1752 NW Market Street, #4419
                  Seattle, WA 98107

Website: rdplegacy.com

ISBN: 978-0-578-24633-8

DEDICATION

This book was published for Robert posthumously, so we dedicate this book to his memory and his desire to tell his story.

We also honor the love and compassion Robert had for people who were suffering for any reason, especially the homeless. Robert's desire was to make a difference in this world, and we pray this book will help to accomplish that.

We pray this book will encourage anyone who is suffering with a mental illness to come out of the shadows and get help, and to tell your stories. You never know who your story will help.

The Palmer Family

WARNING!

This book contains material related to suicide, suicidal ideations, and the graphic description of a suicide attempt.

TABLE OF CONTENTS

FOREWORD

My name is Howard McCrary. I am a Grammy-nominated musician, arranger, composer, singer, and recipient of The ASCAP Duke Ellington Award. It was my great honor to be friends with Robert Palmer. The magnitude of his musical brilliance is beyond description. Our mutual friend Chaka Khan used to describe him as "other", which meant out of this world. Robert had the ability to see and hear from beginning to end songs that did not exist. He could feel the groove for *Changing Faces*, *Time After Time*, and ask, "Did you hear that, bruh?" If I said no, he would say, "It's time for a Manny's break!" Then we'd hop into his sports car and go to Manny's Delicatessen Bakery, to buy sugarless cookies. This alone would give us energy for the next five hours.

I was introduced to Robert by Ms. Ingrid Sunday Wang. She hired me to co-produce a project with her and Robert. We had so many mutual friends and found out we had many things in common, specifically our musical range. That's when I discovered what a genius he was. He invited me to work on many projects with artists like Jennifer Love Hewitt, Sandra St. Victor, and many more. We reached our production partnership's pinnacle when we composed, arranged, and produced Chaka Khan's album, *Come To My House* with the Artist Formerly Known as Prince. We also co-wrote a song Chaka called *Spoon*. Prince loved the way Robert played guitar and commented on his chord progressions, saying, "He's sick with it!"

When I moved to Hong Kong, Robert and I kept in touch. By then Robert had decided to switch careers and become a motivational speaker. His new goal was to mentor and inspire the future players in the music industry. He later told me he was starting to receive information vibrationally that would be confirmed on the internet months later. In my eyes, he was becoming a prophet. He could read your thoughts. I knew him too well to know that he was not joking because I had experienced this phenomenon on many occasions while working in the studio with him.

A little over a year ago, my ex-wife Tammy McCrary arranged a luncheon for us in Los Angeles. I had no idea this would be the last time I would see him. He told me, "For your Parkinson's, Howard, keep taking the Levodopa you've been prescribed, and you will be just fine, bruh." Tammy hadn't told him anything about my prescription! That was our very last encounter.

I had no idea he had been diagnosed with bipolar depression. Robert was a private and proud man. He would never admit he was vulnerable to mental or emotional suffering despite all of his amazing accomplishments. This was heartbreaking news to me and everyone who knew him. The next time a friend asks me for help or reaches out to me through their silent pain, I will be there.

Robert, we love you, and we will be there for your children and family. Your music and your legacy will live forever in our hearts. Thank you for all of your timelessly magnificent music and knowledge.

In loving remembrance,
Howard McCrary

FROM MISERY TO HOPE

PROLOGUE
BY KARY YOUMAN

It was 10 p.m. on Thursday, December 31, 2020. A cloud of sadness came over me as I thought about the many families who had lost their loved ones to COVID-19. I felt blessed that my family and friends had survived this horrible pandemic thus far. My fiancée and I had visited her father and we were on our way to pick up food from the nearby Indian restaurant we love. I received an incoming call from my youngest sister while we were en route.

It had become a family tradition for me, my siblings, and Dad to connect every other Thursday at 6 p.m. via video chat, to catch up and check in with each other. New Year's Eve was no exception. However, Dad wasn't on the call on this particular night. Two weeks prior, he'd declined an invitation to celebrate his sixty-seventh birthday with us because he wasn't feeling well. We all knew he suffered from severe depression and was diagnosed with bipolar depression years ago, so we were aware of his mood swings.

I had a strange feeling and couldn't imagine why she would be calling me back before midnight since we had just spoken. Maybe she forgot to tell me something. Was it a pocket dial? Either way, I had just enough time to answer her call before stepping into the restaurant to grab our food.

"Hello?"

Without hesitation, she said, "Dad's dead..."

It felt like a hot dagger was slowly being pushed into my heart. I was at a loss for words. I told her I would call her back as soon as I got home. I walked into the restaurant to grab our takeout food order and slowly made my way back to the exit. Before I could step outside the restaurant, the cashier said, "Happy New Year, my friend. We made it!" I tried to smile before walking out the door, but I couldn't.

In the sixty seconds it took for me to get back to the car, I kept asking myself, "What else could I have done to help him? Was it my fault? Why did this happen?" I slowly opened the car door. I didn't want to kill the vibe, so I decided to wait until we were home to share the heartbreaking news. I told my fiancée I had a headache and needed to close my eyes for a bit.

My mind was going in circles. During the car ride home, I thought about our first conversation and how meeting him only two years prior had been a life-altering experience. After one year of getting to know each other, mostly over the phone, he decided to relocate to Portland, Oregon (where I live), to start a new chapter in his life. On many occasions, he shared how much he loved living in Oregon and how cultivating a relationship with me and my five other siblings was a dream come true.

His passion for writing and telling stories, and the hours of conversation we had about life, family, mental health, music, and spirituality were the catalysts for this book. I didn't know, nor did I understand, how severe his depression was until he opened up and shared with me how he'd gone *From Misery To Hope*.

PART 1

THE EARLY YEARS

I was born on December 19, 1953, in Cleveland, Ohio. My dad's name, your grandfather, was Robert Lee Palmer, and my mom's name, your grandmother, was Ruthie Dell Palmer. She had five children from a previous marriage. She didn't want me to be a 'junior', so she gave me the middle name, Donnell. My dad was a train mechanic for the Pennsylvania Railroad. He died when I was two, and at the age of five, my two sisters, my mom, and I moved to Oakland, California. We stayed with our grandparents, her mom and stepdad. He was a Baptist minister, so that meant church every Sunday. That was my introduction to God and I've remained a Christian throughout most of my life.

Music started for me when I was introduced to it at the age of ten. I can still remember riding around in Oakland, California, in the early Sixties in my older sister's deep-purple convertible Pontiac, my head leaning back, staring at the starry skies, as the tinny radio blasted out Motown hits by The Supremes, Smokey and The Miracles, The Temptations, etc. You could hear it throughout the neighborhoods. It was intoxicating! From that moment forward, I knew—somehow or someway—I needed to be a part of the magic coming from that radio.

After a few years, we moved from Oakland to a rough and rural part of California. Sixty miles east of Los Angeles, it is called San Bernardino. To this day, it still has the highest murder rate in California. Because of that, when I grew up, a lot of my best friends either wound up in prison for life, murdered, dead from drug overdoses, or in mental institutions. I believe it's one of the reasons I've dealt with a life-long crippling-battle with depression—from trying to make sense of it all at such a young age.

When did music start for me? At the age of thirteen I got my first guitar. Shortly after that I heard Stax Records session guitarist Steve Cropper play on Aretha Franklin's *Chain of Fools*, and later the music of Jimi Hendrix. I played in a band and had to learn most of his songs. This was when I knew this would be my life's path and a possible way out of the horrible place I grew up in.

One day I was expelled from the ninth grade. I can still remember my mother telling me, "You will not become another dead statistic in this town. You need to make something great from a bad situation." Bless her soul and may she rest in peace. Those words still ring true to this very day. I resorted to staying in the house, sitting in my room and practicing until my fingers bled.

By the mid-Seventies I'd had my first child, a beautiful baby girl. It was one of the greatest moments of my life. We all lived together for a while in San Bernardino. It was around this time that the soul pop group WAR signed me and my early childhood friends to our first major record deal (it would have been the equivalent of a half-million dollars today). We were in our early twenties. After a while, the commute became too much for the band, so we all decided to move to Hollywood. Sometimes, we also played at

Vietnam rallies for actress Jane Fonda and comedian Dick Gregory. Those were fun times.

I remember one day in 1975, our band was standing in front of a house on Hollywood Boulevard when this guy walking his dogs stopped and talked to us. We told him we were working on our first album. He said he was an unemployed actor. He had written a script and the movie studio had asked to buy it from him, but they wanted to cast a more well-known actor in the lead. He'd refused because he wanted to play the part himself. We told him that since he was broke he should perhaps consider it. That's when he said, "Never sell your dreams." We never forgot that.

One year later, I was walking past a movie theatre and noticed that same actor on the poster: it was Sylvester Stallone, in the lead role of his movie script *Rocky*. I called the guys over and showed them. We never forgot what he'd said.

Soon after that, my daughter's mom and I separated because she didn't want to move to the Los Angeles area no matter how much I begged her. We just seemed to grow apart after that. I simply didn't know how to deal with the severe bipolar depression that had already taken over. I ran away from everything. I had no coping skills. My daughter really suffered. I saw her less and less because of it and because of the drugs I was taking, and now the alcohol had gotten so bad I began to lose touch with reality and my priorities. That's something I regret to this very day. I can't make that time up to her.

Not long after that, we disbanded. In the late Seventies, I was still living in L.A. and went on to do sessions around the city, playing on records for Natalie Cole, Peabo Bryson, Patti LaBelle, LTD, Robbie Dupree, Bobby Womack, and working on box-office hit movies, such as *Bustin' Loose* (with Richard Pryor and Cicely Tyson) and *Cheech and Chong*. Things had now gotten pretty out of control. I stayed high all the time just to fight it. I had developed a very expensive cocaine habit and was on the verge of financial ruin. I needed to start going to church again, but I didn't. I didn't feel I needed God in my life at that time. I was fine being out of control. It had become my normal.

One day around 1980, I got a call from my good friend, Lawrence Hilton Jacobs from the *Welcome Back, Kotter* show. He asked me to come down for a recording session. When I arrived, I was introduced to a new artist being produced by an NBC executive named Sy Kravitz. His wife, Roxie Roker (the actress from *The Jeffersons*), would drop off their son on her way to film the show. I would give him guitar lessons whenever we broke for lunch. He was a quick learner. That kid was Lenny Kravitz. I ran into him years later in a restaurant in 1997. By then he was a world-famous singer. I told him how proud of him I was. He remembered the story in detail.

It was around this time that I met and soon started dating this amazing woman. Her name was Penny. Life with her was good and we got along well. She would later become my wife. It wasn't long before we were heavily doing drugs, and we eventually lost our apartment. At times, we even slept in our car in alleys.

Between session jobs and touring, most of our money was going on fueling our out-of-control drug and alcohol habits. Every dime of it. We didn't eat half the time just so we could buy drugs. I was touring with Billy Preston at that time and we would open in Las Vegas at The Sahara Hotel for Don Rickles. While at the hotel, we ate like kings—filet mignon, the best champagne money could buy, you name it—and there was always plenty of cocaine... mounds of it.

Every time we'd return to L.A., we were back to sleeping in our car or at a friend's. We were essentially homeless. It was a horrible roller coaster and we just didn't quite know how to get off of it. My depression was at an all-time-low. I always suffered in silence. I never told Penny; I didn't know how.

I clearly remember working one day at a recording session with Bobby Womack, Billy Preston, Johnny Guitar Watson, Eddie Kendricks, and Mitch Mitchell (Jimi Hendrix's drummer). I had done so much cocaine and alcohol that I fell over on the floor right in the middle of the session. I had overdosed. The next thing I knew, I was in the hospital with doctors trying to revive me. That was my first big warning, but it still wasn't enough to make me quit. I needed to be in rehab. Little did we know that fate was waiting just around the corner, and it was clearly beyond anything we could have ever imagined.

A Glimpse of Heaven

The date was April 17, 1985. I was playing with legendary keyboardist Billy Preston at The Sahara Hotel in Las Vegas. We were there again, opening for famed comedian Don Rickles, whom I'd become friends with. Don would always come backstage to wish us a great show just before we went on. Afterward, he'd sometimes have me walk through the casino with him. He'd always tell me the same story, about how back in his early days he was doing comedy in the same hotel, only in a smaller room. Sinatra would come in and see his act. "It was Sinatra who discovered me," he'd always say.

On this particular day, a Monday, I had the day off. Penny and I were invited to a party at a friend's house. I'd gotten high earlier that day, so when I walked outside later that night I dropped just-like-that. I flatlined. I had overdosed from cocaine and alcohol abuse. Everything went black, as if someone had tripped over the plug on a TV and the picture had gone dead. There was darkness, then quiet. Next, there were bright lights and sparkling halos. I had slipped away to a foreign place.

Suddenly, just like that, I was back. I woke up to the sound of unfamiliar voices. I looked around and was sitting on the center console of our sports car. I could now hear Penny's voice to my right. I turned and shouted, "Help me!" She looked at me, and when I saw her expression, my heart stopped and I flatlined again.

The bright lights were back, and there was a strange quiet around me, except the sound of gurgling, like someone was under water. I no longer could feel my body or presence. It had left me. There was no sadness. I was without emotion. I just was. I don't recall the feeling of time passing or any concerns. Was I dead? I had no clue, nor did it matter. The orbs of light were inviting. They were alive as I moved toward them. I was no longer the bearer of thought, just pure consciousness.

The lights suddenly left, and in the next moment Penny was running around, screaming frantically. I was shocked at what I saw. "Penny!" I yelled. She couldn't hear me. There was a paramedic truck, and men were leaning over me as I lay in the rain. One had a defibrillator with paddles, administering shocks to my chest. I could read his lips as he silently shouted, "Clear!" "Hit!" "Clear !" "Hit!" "He still has no pulse!" Sadly, there was still only a flat line. I had gambled one too many times and it had finally caught up with me.

Penny stopped pacing. She grabbed my hand, but I couldn't feel it. I wanted to feel her touch so badly, to let me know I wasn't dead, but I still couldn't feel it! She released it, and it dropped lifelessly off to the side of the gurney. I called out to her, "Penny! I'm still here! I'm still here!" I kept shouting, but she didn't hear me. The paramedics pushed her away. When the truck opened and I saw them putting me in it, a glowing light appeared to close in around me. It came between them and me as the images on the ground began to fade behind the bright lights. They were getting brighter and brighter. The glow was now as bright as the sun, yet I could stare straight into it. If this was a glimpse of heaven, then it was beyond anything I could have described. There was now only light in a vacuum...

I was now being pronounced 'clinically dead' by the paramedics. I'd had a cardio-pulmonary arrest—a heart attack—and total kidney and respiratory failure. I was surrounded by this force of light that brought total calm. It kept getting more intense as I was drawn into it, as if it were pulling me in. Then, suddenly, I was jerked back into myself. I lay on a gurney in the ER with my eyes wide open, wondering what had just happened. When later asked what I'd seen, I told the story to the doctors. They said it was impossible for me to know it because I had been clinically dead with no brain activity at the time. Penny. The paramedics' records confirmed my story about the events I had seen while lying on the gurney in the rain, dead.

I was now on life support and somehow, miraculously, brought back to life. My kidneys were totally destroyed and I had to be put on dialysis. Just when Penny thought things couldn't get any worse for us, she discovered she was five months pregnant! Would the child even survive what she'd gone through? There was a lot going on in our lives at that moment.

Next, the hospital's financial services were on Penny's back about who was paying my increasingly large bill. When Don Rickles heard what had happened to me, he rushed over to the hospital. He told them to do whatever it took to keep me alive. The doctors said, more-than-likely, my kidneys would never come back and a donor might be needed. This was from the years of drug and alcohol abuse.

By this time, most of my family had flown in. They were told that when the doctors had opened me up, three-quarters of my colon had rotted away from gangrene and was floating detached inside my stomach. They didn't even have to cut it out. They just removed it and threw it in the trash. It was destroyed. I'd gambled too many times and finally lost.

After that, I was told by my doctors and nurses that throughout the entire hospital people were talking about this 'miracle man' who God had brought back from the dead; that he and his family must have had a lot of faith. I felt guilty every time I heard that. I'd lie there in my bed every night, crying my eyes out because I knew there were more deserving young kids in there with other life-threatening illnesses who wouldn't have a chance at even making it to a high school prom. There I was, nothing more than a drunk and a drug-addict, who'd thrown his life away, but still I knew it had given a lot of people hope, despite the fact it was eating me alive.

Late one night in my room, I was awakened by a Jamaican woman at the foot of my bed. She was praying and asking God to spare the life of her son, who was down the hall in critical condition. "Please, God, spare my son as you have done for this miracle man here," she prayed. When she noticed I was awake, she asked me, "Please, Mr. Miracle Man, can you ask God to spare my son?"

I was taken aback by her request. "I don't have that kind of power," I told her. "But I will pray for him for you."

"The good Lord has plans for you, that's why He brought you back from the dead," she said.

I found out the next morning her son had died. I was now wondering, *'What is the reason He brought me back? Here I am, an alcoholic and a drug addict. I don't deserve to live over good people who haven't wasted their lives as I have.'*

I prayed to God that night and asked Him what was His purpose for bringing me back. What had I done to deserve it? There were a lot of good people there who deserve it more than I did. *'This poor lady who lost her son, how do You explain that to me? How do You determine Your choices?'* I was no closer in that moment to understanding God's ways than I was before I'd died. How long would it remain a mystery?

In those next few weeks, there were people dying all around me. One minute I was talking to them and the next morning they were dead and had been taken out. There was so much death around me that it was starting to take a toll on my understanding of life.

In those next few months, my family and I prayed harder than at any time of my life. One morning the doctors walked in and stood around my bed with puzzled looks on their faces. I just knew that by the grace of God, our prayers had been answered. One doctor explained that both of my kidneys—after being totally destroyed—had come back at the same moment that morning, which they said was nothing short of a miracle. After what my body had endured in those last few months, there was no way I should have come out alive.

"God must've brought you back for a reason, young man."

Little did he know, I'd seen a small glimpse of heaven while the parallax view of my body struggled to survive. Why? Somehow there was a dark beauty to that question I couldn't understand. But it was far from over, and the most amazing part of it was yet to come.

A New Life

When we left the hospital that day, Penny and I were very grateful to God for my life having been given back to me and her having a healthy pregnancy, despite what she'd gone through. We made a promise to God that we would find a church. We got married. We also removed from our lives all the friends who still did drugs and alcohol. We had zero tolerance for it. Things had now gotten better. We were going to church, and when our daughter China was born, she had complications and almost died, but she was eventually okay.

Things were now great. I was working with Little Richard, and back touring the world with Billy Preston, even living with him in Amsterdam for a period. I was scoring films with a good friend of mine named Mark Davis. I actually got to be in one with Miles Davis (no relation). What an experience that was!

It was now the beginning of the Nineties and my son was born; we named him a junior. Around this time, I still hadn't gotten professional help to deal with an addictive personality, so my addictiveness simply transferred itself somewhere else. Cracks began to appear in our marriage, but instead of going to a marriage counselor I dealt with it through infidelity. I ruined my marriage. I learned a hard lesson from that. I remember calling Penny one day and making a promise to call her every single night—for as long as it took—until she said she was able to move on with her life. I believe it went on for almost a year, until one day she said, "Robert, you know what? I think I'm fine now."

After that night, I vowed never to do that to anyone again, and to this very day I haven't. That was a very sad time I'm not very proud of. Penny ended up moving back to North Carolina with the kids, but that's entirely another story. All I can say is, she's an amazing person who's been through a lot. I have so much respect for her. We're very close to this day. I'd do anything for her, as she has done for me.

The year was now 1994, and I was in the studio producing an album for The Gap Band. Everyone had gone home for the night. As I walked to my car, my arm suddenly felt as if it had been severed. The pain was excruciating. I'd later find out by doctors, that I'd developed severe and debilitating joint inflammation after my body had suffered from years of hard drug and alcohol abuse, kidney failure, and the heart attack. All the joints in my body felt as if they were being crushed by a truck twenty-four hours a day. I was constantly in emergency wards at four o'clock in the morning, taking more opioids, which still didn't ease all of the pain.

Later I was diagnosed with an auto-immune disorder. Some of the best specialists in the field said they'd never seen anything like it in all their years of practice. I was now forced to take higher levels of opioids just to function, which only exacerbated the depression.

"I want out of this life! No one should have to suffer like this," I told my girlfriend.

I was living in a quiet hell every day, which made it hard to work or focus. I had a hard time trying to understand why God had brought me back to life just to suffer this way and hadn't just left me in that beautiful place where I was when I'd died. I began losing my faith at that time.

Despite this, I kept it to myself. My career continued to flourish with number-one records around the world. It was in 1998, one night just before going to bed, that I received a call from Chaka Khan, with whom I'd written some songs just months prior. What a beautiful experience that was. She's such an amazing talent, which I'm sure everyone already knows. She put this gentleman on the phone, and I instantly recognized his voice. It was Prince. He was inviting me to his Paisley Park studios in Minneapolis to work with him, Chaka, and Howard McCrary on her new record, *Come to My House*. Prince and I talked a lot about God and spirituality. The irony was that he also was taking opioids for pain at that time.

In those next few years, I was still in so much pain, which only made the depression worse. I had no choice but to keep driving myself. On the other hand, life would have been great for most. I was working with artists such as Will Downing, Disney pop idol Jesse McCartney, Changing Faces, Lionel Richie, Patti LaBelle, Sheena Easton, The Whispers, Deniece Williams, Jennifer Love Hewitt, Avant, and Hilary Duff, just to name a few. I worked on a number of box office hit films: *A Cinderella Story* (with Hilary Duff and Regina

King), *Deep Blue Sea* (with Samuel Jackson), and countless others.

In 2005, I co-wrote the hit record *Stickwitu* for the Pussycat Dolls. The album would go on to sell 9 million records, making it the eighth biggest selling girl group record of all time. The song also went on to be nominated at the 2006 Grammys and the 2006 Soul Train Music Awards. It went platinum in the U.S., and sold three million in the world. In January of 2006, it went to #1 on The Billboard charts, and #1 on the World Airplay Chart as well. It entered the chart at #1 in the U.K., dethroning Madonna, who had held it for weeks. I signed a nice publishing deal with Sony/ATV publishing, the biggest publishing company in the world. In 2006, I was awarded the prestigious BMI award for songwriters.

It wasn't the success I was worried about. I felt empty and without a purpose other than creating music. Somehow, I knew there was more spiritually I could be a part of. Yet without notice, after having such a big hit, the pressure for my writing partners and I to duplicate our success was now upon us. My phone was ringing off the hook from all over the world with requests to write hits for other artists. As a result, I had an anxiety attack so bad I wanted to die. The added burden was overwhelming. Strange as it may seem, it wasn't so much the pressure of coming up with more hits but the added depression that always tagged alongside me. I simply couldn't take it anymore. Success had now become an insidious, growing monster.

In 2009 I decided I could no longer bear the combined disorders any more—the depression, the suicidal thoughts and the chronic-pain disorder. After months of contemplation, I decided to isolate myself from the industry, and even family and friends, and try and get a hold on my life. By this time, I was losing so much money due to mismanagement that I was now in total financial ruin. I got rid of the big house and scaled down to a medium-size one. Within a few years, the IRS had cleaned out the rest of my savings. I had spiraled so out of control, mentally and financially, that there was nothing left. The disorders had robbed me of everything. I then scaled down to a small one-bedroom apartment. It was now the lowest point in my life since the heart attack.

THE NDE

The year was 2010, and after a year of self-imposed isolation from the world, I reached out to a few friends. I even started to talk about doing music again. I didn't mention the problems that still lingered. The chronic debilitating pain had gotten worse, along with the depression.

This is when things began to get very strange. I was starting to experience electromagnetic anomalies. My razor in the morning on a full charge would drain the moment I turned it on. Light bulbs in rooms would constantly flicker when I walked in. My cell phone volume would go up and down when I picked it up. I walked outside one night and used my phone to film myself walking to a streetlight and standing underneath it for a few minutes. Suddenly, it cut off. When I backed up, the light came back on. I repeated it at least four times. I still have that video. It was pretty amazing.

My friends were starting to notice it as well. The more it happened, the more they brought it to my attention. One day, a very close friend was emailing me some info when he ended the message, talking about his diabetes. Out of nowhere, I hypothesized about what was causing it. He responded with a question mark. I didn't know what had prompted me to say what I'd told him. A few weeks later, an article in a popular science and health website stated that after testing mice, researchers believed they were making new progress in finding one of the contributing factors to diabetes. It was exactly what I had shared with my friend in that email. There was no way I could have known that. When I sent him the email a few days later, he responded: "WOW!!! OK, this falls in the unbelievable category. You are going to have to document your theories and get 'em out to the public. Astounding, my brotha, simply astounding!"

On another occasion, back in September of 2011, I told a good friend of mine who had worked in the medical field for over thirty years that I had a crazy hypothesis about why organ donor transplant rejection occurs so frequently. It just came out of nowhere in a conversation that was totally unrelated. I think my friend was taken aback by my sudden abruptness. It was primitive, but I essentially said that if doctors first made sure the organ of the donor's circadian rhythm (which is run by the suprachiasmatic nucleus in the brain) was in sync before performing the transplant, the rejection rate might be lowered considerably. Months later, I found a paper that had been submitted based on that same hypothesis.

These kinds of strange events were now happening quite frequently for no reason, to the point where I needed to get some answers and advice. It was on a Thursday afternoon when I searched the internet for experts in the field of Near Death Experiences (NDEs) to see if there was a connection of some sort. After enough research, I was directed to a book titled, *Coming Back to Life,* by a woman named P.M.H. Atwater. I picked it up later that week. Once I started reading it I couldn't put it down. She said she'd had several NDEs when she was younger. Everything that was happening to me was in the exact sequential order as in her book. The similarities were astounding.

Atwater said some of the symptoms she'd experienced were signs of deep depression, isolation from friends, and heightened intuition. I knew who would call, text, or send an email before it happened. I would do it with them just as they were about to contact me at that very second. Friends had begun to notice as well, and commented several times on the frequency of it.

One day, my eleven-year-old daughter was watching TV. I was looking in the other direction, toward the wall, talking to my sister on the phone. Suddenly, everything I was saying to my sister, appeared on the TV (the exact image of it) at moment. It even interrupted the current show that was on. My daughter yelled out each time it happened, and my sister overheard her. This happened twice in a row. Neither she nor my daughter could believe what they were hearing. It appeared to be telekinetic. Who knows?

Later that year, I joined an NDE webslte. It was very comforting being able to talk to people in a community all over the world who had experienced some of the same phenomena. It was called IANDS (International Association for Near Death Studies). Their stories about some of the after-effects they'd experienced were sequentially almost identical to mine. It was amazing. What really struck me were the similarities in the visions of heaven when we were out of our bodies.

There were so many great people I communicated with from that society. They were always very supportive, but within a short time I drifted away and lost touch with most of them. It was unfortunate for me that I had deeper issues to deal with, which I knew they couldn't help me with—chronic pain, depression, and thoughts of suicide.

When my mother first heard about what was happening she thought I was crazy—until I told her things in detail. She said there was no way I could have known because I hadn't been born when they had happened. I described a room she was sitting in while feeding one of my older sisters who'd just been born. There was a varnished radio to her right with the mesh grill... the colors of the quilt she was sitting on... she said she'd never told me that.

My older brother was sick with terminal prostate cancer and multiple sclerosis. I was glad I had gotten a chance to speak to him before he fell into a coma. One night I was lying on my sofa when a freezing cold air came over me. It was very warm outside, so it was unusual. I saw a vision of my brother hovering above me, saying, "Robert, tell Mother I'm okay." He showed me his hands and arms, and said he was better now. I just knew it was some kind of dream or something, but it reminded me of that beautiful place I had gone to when I'd died. Oh, how I wanted to go back there so badly!

That morning, my sister called me, and before she said anything, I told her what had happened the night before and what he'd said to me. She was stunned, confirming he had died in the night. I shared with my mother what he'd said to tell her. She cried and said she felt comforted by it. By this point, after the things I had shared with her, I'm sure she believed me now that this gift was real.

The night Whitney Houston died, my sister called. I told her, on that coming Saturday, they would bury Whitney in a gold casket and a purple robe. That Saturday she was buried in that exact casket and robe. By now my sister was getting used to it. I was coming to understand that on April 1985, the night I had died and crossed over, I had glimpsed heaven. I was now sure of it.

I needed to get answers for some of the other strange anomalies that were occurring. I reached out to a renowned expert on the subject, named Bruce Greyson. I didn't expect him to respond to my cmail, but within hours, he did. His knowledge about NDEs really helped me because by this point I was desperate to know what was causing it. Greyson made sense of some of the phenomena possibly associated with it. From his research, which went back to the early Eighties, he'd interviewed thousands of cases. There were a lot of similarities with theirs and my own. He had a lot of questions for me about some of the other anomalies that were happening. I even sent him the video of me walking under the streetlight that flickered on and off.

This was now beginning to take a toll on me. I didn't want it anymore. It was a curse. What did I need it for? I was a person who was constantly on the verge of suicide. I was a wreck. "God, please give it to someone that will put it to good use. I'm just not that one."

One morning on November 3, 2012, I was meditating. Two hours into it, I had a vision of a Catholic priest or saint who came to me and said his name was St. Martin. He was black with short, cropped hair. He had on a long white frock. His facial features were very distinct and clear. It was strange because I wasn't Catholic, and in my limited knowledge of Catholicism I had never heard of a black priest or saint. I didn't know the name of any, other than the popular ones, like St. Peter, St. Paul, St. Luke. Why was he coming to me in a vision?

I immediately went over to the computer to look him up. When the screen opened to his name St. Martin de Porres in Wikipedia, a picture came up with his life story. I pushed away from the computer in amazement and shock. He was the man who had come to me in the vision; the exact same features. The Wikipedia entry said he became a saint when it was verified he had been seen in three places at once. He died in 1639 on November 3, the very date I was sitting there and reading it. It was beyond believable. He was fifty-nine when he died. What could this possibly be saying to me? The number fifty-nine and St. Martin de Porres?

Later that night, I called my sister Gloria to tell her. She thought it was pretty amazing! Especially that he'd died on the same day I'd seen him. She would be the only one I told that story to, until years later when it would make a connection spiritually, and enlighten someone's life—in the most unusual of places.

Why had I been given this gift?

THE BROKEN THREAD, PART 1

New Year's Eve, 2012, for me was very uneventful. I just stood in the window of my apartment and listened to the festivities going on outside in my neighborhood. I didn't feel motivated to be part of them. I was back at that low point again and wasn't sure if I'd make it out this time.

I was finding more and more reasons not to live. Why go on? Why prolong the agony? These were questions that were seared in my mind like a freshly branded calf. I found depression to be something quite elusive. It always seemed to show up in time to invade whatever semblance of happiness I tried to garner. And it was winning the fight. Suicide was heavier on my mind than ever before, and that's when I made the hard decision.

As humans, we tend to gravitate toward similarities. I noticed that suicides were beginning to happen quite frequently amongst people in the entertainment industry. For example, Don Cornelius and Tony Scott (the brother of Ridley Scott, the film director/producer) both committed suicide in 2012. Tony Scott, who was the English director and producer of *Beverly Hills Cop II* and *Top Gun*, jumped off the San Pedro bridge.

DAY 1...

After all those years of threatening to commit suicide, I was finally prepared to go through with it. The day I officially chose was May 3, 2013. I had two days left to plan it out. Nothing mattered at this point because I wasn't going to be around in three days to have to worry about it, or anything else for that matter. I went through my belongings and pictures, and separated them into envelopes for my family. It was eerie, but I told myself there would be no turning back this time. I would follow through. I couldn't remove the thought that I was going to die on May 3rd—gone from this earth by my own hands.

I went online, trying to decide which way I would do it. There were hundreds of possibilities, but the only problem was I didn't have access to the materials for most of them. This limited it to three choices: hanging, cutting my wrists, or using a gun. After a few hard and painful hours, I finally narrowed it down: I would cut my throat and wrists. If that didn't work, I'd go down to the bridge over the San Pedro River and jump off.

I went into the kitchen and looked at the knife block. I chose five large butcher knives, reached up over the top of the fridge, and pulled down the sharpener. I took the knives into the living room and sat down on the floor, beneath the window. I could hear the last of the rush-hour traffic in the distance, horns blaring, and the smell of someone cooking dinner as I began to sharpen each one, over and over again until they were razor-sharp. It was now evening and the silhouette of the moon illuminated through the window, providing the only light in the room. I continued to sharpen the knives like a madman as they glistened in the moonlight.

What goes through one's mind at such a grim and decisive moment? The only thing I can say is 'regret'. My list of regrets was so long it would probably fill the Library of Congress. Just then, I was startled by the ringing of my cell. It was my sister. We had an amazing relationship. She was my 'rock' and would take it pretty hard if she knew what I was planning to do, so I didn't answer her call. I just let it go to voicemail.

After such a grueling day I was getting sleepy. I was trying to fill my mind with things of substance and not waste precious minutes on mind chatter. I tried to keep my eyes open, but to no avail. I couldn't fight it any longer; I was sleepy. Within minutes, I found myself falling asleep on the floor beneath the window sill for the night. I now had two days left to live.

DAY 2...

I woke up that morning and wiped the sleep from my eyes. I looked around the floor, viewing the knives I realized I'd forgotten to put away before going to bed. It was numbing to see them that early. I gathered them up from the floor and spent hours pacing back and forth.

Every few minutes, I stopped to catch my breath. My breathing had gotten heavier as my thoughts were now racing uncontrollably, like someone in a stolen car breaking through a police barricade. '*Slow down!*' I said to myself. '*Everything will soon be okay.*' This is probably a normal reaction at this point for anyone attempting suicide. Unfortunately, those who have been successful aren't around to talk or write about their experiences—or to help walk me through mine.

I walked over and sat on the sofa, grabbing my King James Bible off the small table near it. I thumbed through it until I reached the book of Proverbs, and read the entire book. In all my years of reading Proverbs I had never understood it—I had simply extrapolated from it. It was such a profound read. For the first time in my life, I truly understood what it was conveying. I asked myself, '*Why did it take until now to understand this book with this level of clarity?*' Maybe my awareness was heightened by the situation at hand.

After that, I went on with my day as usual. Surprisingly, I didn't have a proverbial 'bucket list' of things to do before I died. If I did, it wouldn't have mattered anyway. My 'bucket' was already filled to the brim with despair, and there was no room left for anything else.

I entered my recording studio to listen to a collection of ideas I'd been working on over the past few months. Running my hands across the knobs on the mixing console, I just wanted to feel the energy from it one last time. This was where it had all started some forty-five years previously. Now, it felt like nothing more than a faded memory of days past, and times I didn't want to remember. After all, this had once been my life. I was still waiting for a sign from God to abort the mission, *any* kind of sign to keep from killing myself. I took a walk outside and prayed on it several times, but nothing came back.

Coming back to the apartment, I sat down on the sofa and exhaled as I told myself, 'This time tomorrow, I won't be alive.' Just the mere thought of it ran a chill up my spine. Was it too late to change my mind? Unfortunately, yes. I knew the tide of nerves I needed to pull this off was now higher than it had ever been before. I wanted to catch it before it ebbed. Unlike all the other times before, I was now ready to step over the line of reason and take that journey into the unknown.

As a kid, during my grandfather's sermons, I'd heard that if you committed suicide you would go to hell. Whether it was true or not, only time would tell. I still got on my knees and asked God's forgiveness for what I was about to do the next day. I went to bed early that night.

The Broken Thread, Part 2

Today was officially *THE DAY*. It didn't feel different to any other day... yet. I didn't want anything to change my mind at this point, so I went back to bed and stayed there until dusk. After a few hours, I got up, walked over to the window and looked out one last time. I headed for the bathroom and was now sitting on the floor, surrounded by knives. Fear and relief permeated the room. I got up and trudged into the living room, the weight of my slippers feeling like steel-toed workmen's boots. I wanted to see if the sun had fully gone down. It had, and the moon was a repeat of the night before, casting ominous silhouettes that appeared to be dancing on the walls.

It was now eight o'clock, and I kept going from the bathroom to the living room, pacing and pacing like a new dad waiting in a delivery room. "Lord, forgive me, for I know not what I do," I mumbled as I resumed the position on the bathroom floor again. I looked at the knives that were arranged in a neat row, wondering which one would get the honor. It was as if they were tiny soldiers lined up as a firing squad. I randomly picked one up, and ever so lightly, slid it across my wrist without breaking the skin. The cold metal against it felt foreign; it was obtrusive. Quickly, I laid it back down on the floor with others.

The sound of someone running a bath upstairs was inviting, if nothing more than a momentary distraction. The sound of birds chirping on my balcony just before sleep told me some things were still fighting to live, that life would still be in the air somewhere long after I was gone. It all represented a vast contrast to the dismal backdrop in the bathroom. I thought about my loved ones and friends one last time, before I slipped off into the waiting arms of that cold abyss of silence we call death.

Nine o'clock. It was time! I made my choice of which knife to use. It took a few minutes before I picked it up. I just stared at it as I sat on the floor. I finally picked it up and drew it closer to my wrist. I closed my eyes and held my head back in the air as I drew it closer and still closer. I took in a deep breath and held it tightly, like a mother holding her child for dear life as it dangled from a cliff. I exhaled as the blade came in contact with my wrist. It felt like a plane hitting the runway tarmac. Slowly I pressed. Then I pressed harder.

Suddenly, out of nowhere, I jumped up from the floor and ran out the bathroom, dropping the knife. My senses were jolted as it hit the floor.

I just can't do it this way! I kept yelling in my head, over and over.

I ran into the living room, and with my back against the wall, I slid down to the floor like a fireman sliding down a pole going to a three-alarm fire—only this blaze was fiercely raging in my head as I began to unravel mentally. I just sat there, gasping for precious air stolen like a thief during a carjacking. Disheveled, I quickly ran toward the kitchen to find my keys.

'Where are they? In the office? Yeah, that's where they are!'

I ran into the office and grabbed them off the desk, then opened the front door and slowed my pace to a creep. I walked down the hallway, my mind racing from fear. I had now decided on plan B. Walking down the two flights of stairs, I paused in the stairwell to ask myself, *'Is this what you really want to do?'*

Finally, I made it to the side door that led to the parking lot. With adrenaline high and palms sweaty, I slowly turned the knob. My hand slipped off. I grabbed it again and walked outside into the brisk night air. As I walked toward my car, I remembered I'd forgotten my wallet with my license in it. *'How will they know who I was if I jump off the bridge without me leaving my driver's license on the car seat?'*

That was part of the plan. Sticking to it, I turned around, went back to the side door, and inserted the key. It wouldn't open. I now felt a panic attack coming. This one was unlike any I'd ever encountered. It was seismic. I stood there, shaking like the branches on a tree just before a Tsunami hits. As the tension mounted, I jiggled the key so hard it almost broke off in the lock. Finally, I stopped, turned around, and walked down the sidewalk along the parking lot. Where was I going? I thought I recognized my neighbor Candice coming toward me.

"Are you okay, Robert?" she asked, a concerned look on her face.

I tried to answer, but couldn't get a word out. I just stood there and stuttered, "Ca-ca-ca-ca..." I was trying to ask her if she could drive me to the hospital. I could tell she didn't understand me but knew something was seriously wrong. I believe I had just frightened her half to death, judging by the look on her face as she walked backwards, almost tripping as she tried to get away. I couldn't go back to the apartment. I just couldn't bear to walk back into the horrid scene that awaited me there.

I walked along the sidewalk, staring at rows of dark apartments. Most of the blinds were closed; I assumed most people had gone to bed already. Knowing my small window of opportunity was still open and that the high tide of nerves required could ebb at any moment, I took advantage of it before that happened. If I missed it, it could take years for me to get it back again.

Right at that moment I noticed at the very end of the neat row of apartments that one still had the lights on. I ran toward it. The feeling of panic had a grip on me like a bear caught in a hunter's trap. All that was going through my mind was, *'I want to kill myself.'* Those words were going around and round in my head, like a carousel full of screaming kids trying to get off after a circuit malfunctions. What I was now experiencing was the broken thread.

THE ABYSS

I walked up to the balcony and could see there was a woman inside. She looked to be attending someone who was paralyzed and lying in a bed. She was white and in her early sixties. I slowly approached their balcony, trying hard not to startle them, knowing my profile of a bald, black man would cause concern, especially at that time of night. I yelled out to her that I lived in the building and couldn't get in because my key didn't work. I shouted out the names of the building managers—Sherry and Wendy—in hopes she would believe me. She kept yelling for me to go away.

I was now at a point on the suicide meter I'd never reached before. It was peaking. I kept telling her I needed help and I needed to get back in the building. Suddenly, the lady disappeared. I stood there in the cold silence, praying to God to let me hurry and end this without dragging it out. I looked around for her. Then, there she was, at the end of the building. She was hanging out the door, yelling for me to come in and to get away from her balcony.

Without thinking, I jumped over her balcony wall, opened the sliding screen, and walked in. Her son was lying there in the bed paralyzed, staring at me like I was some madman off the streets— which at this point, I probably was. I remember I kept saying to him, "I'm not going to hurt you! I'm not going to hurt you!"

As I left the bedroom and headed for the front of her apartment, she came running back in, screaming at the top of her lungs for me to get out. Calmly, I told her over and over, "I'm not here to hurt you. I just want to kill myself." I kept trying to convince her.

"No, you can't kill yourself!" she responded.

I told her, "I have to. There's no way out for me."

She pointed her finger to the open door. 'Why don't you go to God?" she yelled.

I responded, "I already have."

She then said, "Why don't you go to your own apartment and do it?"

I walked over to the front door of the small apartment, shut it, then went into her kitchen, which was right next to it, and searched for knives. There were two small knives on the counter. The woman opened the door again and yelled repeatedly for me to leave.

What am I doing? The question that kept going through my head. Finally, I closed my eyes and slid the knife across my wrist. There was no blood. I applied more pressure. Nothing. Not a drop! I searched the room for a sharper knife, maybe a butcher knife. I spotted a knife block on the counter filled with an assortment of them. She was getting more hysterical by the minute. I walked over and reached for several knives, assuring her I wasn't going to harm her or her family. I gave her my word, but what did that mean? This poor woman had never seen me in her life.

I went back to the countertop, closed my eyes again and pressed harder. I kept applying pressure until I felt a burning sensation. I'd finally broken through the skin! The blood was flowing as I raised the knife and started a new cutting area. It started bleeding as well. I was lost inside the act and wanted to hurry up and get it over with.

At that moment, it seemed as if everything was in slow motion. Her voice sounded slurred like a sloweddown record. The knife slitting my wrist was painful. I could feel the warm blood running down my arm. As it ran from the two cuts, like fresh river streams in a backwoods lake, I was at the point-of-no-return. I picked up another knife, hoping it would be sharper. I raised it to my throat and started slicing. I sliced and sliced in a stroking motion—almost as if I were a violinist, bowing it frantically at the peaking end of a concerto, titled, *An Opus for the Disturbed*. Unfortunately, there wasn't a standing ovation from the solo audience, just sheer shock and terror as I added more pressure with each new stroke.

The blood was now running between my fingers. Suddenly, I stopped. I couldn't do this in front of her. I ran to her bathroom. I tried locking the door, but the lock was stuck and it took a minute of wrestling with it to finally get it locked. I stood there, staring in the mirror at a person I didn't know any more—maybe had never known at all. I was just another one of God's lost sheep who had wandered out the fence of His protection, beyond the gates of sanity.

I then noticed the silence of the lady's apartment. Her voice was no longer screaming from the other side of the door in the hall begging me not to do it. I stood there, wondering what I'd just done. Could I finish what I'd started? The continued silence from the other side of the door was haunting. Where had she gone? Minutes had passed. The blood was now running down her sink onto the bathroom floor.

'*Maybe she went to call the police,*' I thought. If that was the case, I now had to make a plan C. If the police came, maybe I could resist arrest, and when I opened the door, they would shoot me. That was the perfect solution. Now all I had to do was stand there and wait. I waited and waited as the warm blood continued to stream down.

I heard noise in the room, coming closer and closer. I could hear what sounded like officers talking. '*Finally,*' I thought. I bit my lip and held it tightly between my teeth as I waited for them to call me to come out. That poor woman. I had come into her place and disrupted her and her son's lives, possibly forever.

"Drop the knife, sir, and come out with your hands in the air!" These were the words I was waiting for. The thought of being shot in the next few minutes was very dark, but I was determined to see it through. He repeated the command and I still didn't respond. I wanted to make sure I had angered them enough, that when I opened the door and lunged at them, it would make them shoot me in defense. But that plan wasn't meant to be. I heard him tell his partner, "When he opens the door, if he hasn't dropped the knife, let's Taser him." I didn't want to be Tasered.

It was all over. Time to give up the attempt. Leaning against the bathroom door, I told them I would comply. I looked in the mirror one last time as I took a deep breath, bracing myself to enter into a brand new world where I'd never been before.

THEY CALLED IT A 5150

I was handcuffed and escorted from the apartment out onto the sidewalk. The night air was brisk and I was freezing. Everywhere you looked, there were curious people in robes and house slippers, all wondering what had happened. I was blinded by the flashing lights of news reporters, all vying for the latest story.

'Now that the thread has finally broken, what happens from here?' That was my question. It felt like a seismic earthquake, on the San Andreas Fault line, had just gone off in my head, releasing the pressure that had built up in it for years.

They finally decided which car would take me. Two sheriffs escorted me to their waiting squad car. We stood there as they conferred before getting in. I could smell the scent of lavender in the air. The night captured the sound of kids skateboarding in the distance.

"Hey, Sheriff, these cuffs are way too tight!" I yelled out. They didn't even respond. He just put me in the backseat and we sped away into the abyss, heading down the road of uncertainty.

I sat there, wrist and throat bleeding, thinking; 'God, what has happened to my life? I can't believe what I just did! My spirit feels so lost right now and I'm scared I'll never get it back. My suicide attempt has failed, and now I have to still be here on this earth to face the consequences of those actions. It wasn't supposed to end like this!' I kept thinking all the way to the mental ward.

One of the officers was calling it in. "Hello, this is Officer Johnson. We're northbound on Valencia Ave to the Emergency ward at the hospital. We've got a 5150 (involuntary psychiatric hold), an attempted suicide. A black male, medium built, approximately fifty-nine years old. Lacerations to both wrists and neck. ETA around fifteen minutes. Over!"

We arrived at the emergency ward, where they bandaged my cuts. Two male nurses finally entered the draped cubicle with a wheelchair and helped me into it.

"Where are we going?" I asked them, concerned and paranoid.

"You'll be just fine, Mr. Palmer. Just please try to relax."

They wheeled me out of the ER, away from the bright lights to an area that was dimly lit. We wound through the back of the building until we finally came to a remote area. It looked very nondescript. We approached a metal door with wire mesh in the small glass area. It looked like a scene out of the movie *Girl Interrupted*. They pushed the buzzer and we waited patiently for someone to come.

After a few minutes, a man wearing thick-rimmed glasses, a lab coat the color of a blue latex glove, and a net over his hair opened the large metal door and the nurses wheeled me inside. I noticed the halls were painted an elementary-school tan and looked very sterile. There was no visible way out as the door locked behind us. It closed with a hollow thud, like the vacuum door to a space capsule. It had reminded me of a lab in a *Frankenstein* horror movie classic.

For the first time in my life I was now in a mental ward. It was very creepy. I had no clue what to expect, except for what I'd seen in movies. *One Flew Over the Cuckoo's Nest* came to mind. It truly had that look to it. They wheeled me into a room where they asked me a million questions. After what seemed the first hundred, I was so exhausted I couldn't answer anymore. I needed a bed and quickly. The place was quiet. I felt like the only patient there, probably due to the enforced curfew, I imagined.

After hours of questioning, we were finally finished. Another night nurse came in to escort me to my room. She was demure in stature and very nice. We walked down several halls, passing rooms that all had faded mint-green-colored doors. They were cracked slightly open, maybe so that they could keep an eye on the patients. They had me undress and gave me an open-back hospital-type gown to wear; then I was shown to my room. It resembled a combination of an insane asylum, a halfway house, and something else that I'm at a loss to describe. There were two twin beds in it; one was pristinely made up. A guy was sleeping in the one closest to the door. The furnishings were sparse, just the bare essentials.

Now that I was there, did I feel like a mental patient? What was it supposed to feel like? I wasn't sure yet, but I still wanted to die—whether I was mental or not, regardless of an evaluation. Did that label me as crazy? (I thought someone who really wanted to die wouldn't be concerned with what label society might place on him or her) I knew I sure wasn't; it was the least of my worries. Finding a way to commit suicide was still at the top of my to-do list.

I looked around the room trying to acquaint myself with my sparse new surroundings, maybe search for a way to finish what I'd started. I was sure that finding a way to break out of this place would be close to impossible, especially when it was designed to hold people like me.

"Where's God?" I wondered. I'd been all the way to hell, and, as far as I was concerned, I was still there. I was quite convinced it was He who had thwarted my plans. Maybe He'd brought me this low to get my attention. If that was the case, He had definitely, without a doubt, succeeded. I prayed for Him to please give the woman and her son comfort after I disrupted their lives, probably forever. I couldn't imagine what they were going through at that moment. More than likely they had been traumatized.

My roommate woke up as I pulled back the bedding. He introduced himself as Raymond and he immediately began telling me about his entire life on drugs. *'It is way too late in the night for this,'* I thought. I just wanted to sleep; it had been a long day. Getting into the bed, I noticed the crisp whiteness of the sheets as I fluffed the down pillow. It was the only thing in the room that reminded me of the five-star hotels I'd once stayed in during my days on the road touring. I could feel the discrete cameras everywhere. It reminded me of some sort of reality show, one about the exploitations of the mentally challenged. This was all new for me.

A few minutes later, a man with a calm voice came over the intercom announcing late night meds. I asked my roomie where to go. He walked me over to the hallway and a door with the top half open, where patients formed a line to receive their medication. Skittles, I called them. I joined the line to get mine.

There was a host of fascinating colors in my Dixie cup, but not as colorful as the scene in the line of people waiting to get theirs. The nurses stood and watched you take every one of them. There were all kinds of people in it, mostly kids who were cutters. I couldn't understand how children so young had no zest for life. It was fascinating to see. They probably looked at me and wondered how a middle-aged man, who had been depressed all his life, could let it go on for so long before finally doing something about it. Could the staff in here really save us from ourselves?

About an hour later, after returning to my bed, my suicidal feelings returned, along with a host of other disturbing psychological thoughts. The chronic pain in my joints was now back. *'I thought the meds were supposed to fix all of that?'* Maybe it takes time for them to work. I still felt extremely suicidal.

I went into the bathroom, out of sight from the cameras, and got on my knees. Behind the industrial-type toilet was a shiny chrome steel fitting. I leaned down and began smashing my head into it incessantly. I did it until I saw blood streaming from my forehead. It swelled profusely, the skin broke, and it was very painful. I went back into the bedroom; Raymond had left temporarily. I banged my head even harder into the cement floor until I blacked out.

A Padded Room

When I came to the next morning, I was still sad. I simply just didn't want to be alive anymore. Was that too much to ask? I had nothing to offer myself, and even less to society. There simply had to be more to life than hit records and success. I didn't want to live with that person anymore. The meds were now making me sleepy. I lay down as the blood dripped from my forehead onto the fresh crisp linen. I was drained and disappointed that I had to live another day.

"Rise and shine! Rise and shine! The director's voice echoed as she walked down the hallway, shouting from room to room for us to get up for breakfast then participate in activities. As I lay there with last night's dried blood sticking my face to the pillow, I knew this wasn't for me. Another director returned after a few minutes and announced it was mandatory. I went to the room and saw that it was filled with patients all playing games. I tried to participate but couldn't get into it because of my social anxiety disorder.

I left and went back to my room to contemplate how I would get out of there and finish the job. There were people everywhere in the halls. Some were standing and banging their heads into the wall. Others were pacing the floor back and forth, head back in the air, screaming at the top of their lungs, until guards came to restrain them. Some were following me for no reason. One middle-aged blonde woman, with runny mascara and unkempt hair, walked by me, opened her robe, flashed her breasts at me and smiled. She had a blank stare on her face. There was so much going on in the halls that I couldn't process it all. It was way too shocking.

Out of nowhere I had a bad panic attack. I felt the walls closing in around me and needed to get out. I couldn't take it. I didn't want to be around anyone. They called security to make sure I was all right. They came running from every direction. Finally, they calmed me down, threatening to put me in a straitjacket if I did it again. I was becoming more agitated and distraught. They had me sit in a chair right in front of a little padded booth with its door wide open. It was intimidating. There was a bed with a straitjacket on it. It was haunting, as if the bed was waiting for its next victim.

They called me in for more evaluations. I was now sitting across the table from a man with a strong African accent. He spoke slowly and precisely. He was a very dark-skinned gentleman, balding and middle-aged. He asked me questions that took me way back to my childhood. It was painful. I tried being evasive, but somehow he managed to corral my thoughts. He reeled them back inside the fence as if he were a cowboy lassoing a calf and rescuing it from the barbed wire it was tangled in. He made a lot of sense, but the sad thing was I didn't want him to make sense. I still wanted to kill myself. I still wanted the cold, abysmal silence. Nothing had changed—or was going to any time soon.

It was obvious he could tell that even his wonderful work as a clinician was losing ground fast with me. I was a hopeless case. "Okay, we're done here, Mr. Palmer," he said as he shook my hand and escorted me out of his office. I turned around just as I got to the door, looked at him, and told him how good I thought he was at his profession. I was just the wrong patient for him to waste his precious time and expertise on. His last words to me were, "You stay here as long as you like, Mr. Palmer. There is no rush. Your wellbeing is the main thing that's important to us."

For some reason, it felt comforting to know that. Later that night, I started to think about life after the mental ward. I drew a blank. I wasn't clear about my life in general. "Where do I go from here? Will my life ever get back to normal? Where will I live? How will my friends respond when I tell them what happened?" These were all questions that haunted me throughout the night as I lay in my bed, restless and unable to sleep.

"Rise and shine! Rise and shine!" echoed the director's voice again the next morning as she went down the hallway, shouting from room to room for us to get up and participate in the activities that were now in progress.

There was a young patient in the group who was around nineteen. He just sat in the corner and wouldn't respond to anything the director was telling him. He was on heavy meds. They said he was always by himself with his back turned to everyone; it was part of his severe disorder. They had tried everything, but had given up after a while. I myself really didn't want to be there, but something in me felt sorry for the kid, so I asked him what his favorite song was. He didn't respond. I tried again, no response. A girl in the group blurted out, "Jamie's favorite song is *Hotel California* by the Eagles." I thought, *'Oh well, what do I have to lose by picking up the guitar and playing it for him. He probably won't turn around anyway, poor kid.'*

I started playing, and some of the kids sang along. Jamie suddenly turned around with a big smile, came over, sat next me, and started singing. "Welcome to the Hotel California..." He almost brought me to tears. The director and the other kids stared at him in amazement.

After everyone in the room cleared out, the director came over to me, still in shock, and said, "His parents won't believe what happened. Wow! He's never participated before." She couldn't wait to tell them. "Why don't you lead the group?" she asked me. I told her I would think about it.

When I returned to my room, I sat on my bunk, closed my eyes, and told God I knew it was He who had touched that kid's spirit. That night in the hallway I ran into Jamie, and despite being heavily sedated I could now see a ray of light with a smile attached to it, trying to break through the dark cloud that held his spirit captive.

"Robert, that was fun. Do you know anymore Eagles songs?" he asked me.

"I can probably remember a few," I told him.

He smiled and continued walking down the hall. Within a few hours, I heard him yelling out in the night, while security tried to secure him from hurting himself, threatening to put him back in the padded room.

Three days had now passed and I was just starting to get acquainted with the facility. It wasn't so bad after all. Maybe I could be the musical director for the kids while I was there. Maybe it was the well-deserved break I'd needed my entire life. Maybe I'd been on the conveyor belt of success too long. Whatever it was, I felt relaxed for the first time. I had no cares in the world.

They really took care of me, despite the fact that my anxiety sometimes came back with a vengeance. Unfortunately, it was then back to them threatening to put me in the padded room. For the most part, I just tried to stay out of everyone's way and keep under the radar — until one morning, the director came running in the room, insisting I come out to the hallway and sign the release form in his hand. I was confused.

I followed him out into the hallway. He took the paper and held it to the wall and pointed to where I was to sign. I was even more confused now, but I took the pen anyway and signed it, without having a chance to read it. He then insisted I had to leave at that minute as he walked me to the door. He opened it wide, and to my disbelief, standing there were at least five sheriffs.

"Are you Robert Palmer?" one of them asked.

"Yes, I am."

"You're under arrest!"

"For what?"

"False Imprisonment!" one of the sheriffs said. "They'll let you know more when you get to jail."

"To *jail*?" I yelled out. "Which one are we going to?"

"You're being transported to the L.A. Men's County Jail," he said. He radioed in, letting them know I was now being transported and would arrive within the hour.

'What have I done to wind up in the L.A. County Jail?' I thought. *I know I went into their home, but these are serious charges against me.*

As we passed the L.A. skyline, I looked out over it. It held no interest anymore. I used to marvel at it whenever I saw it. Now, it was no more than a clustered nebula of blurred lights, reflecting the smog of L.A. I wanted to die even more now, especially knowing they were taking me to jail. I wouldn't survive there, I'd always said. I'm not jail material.

After riding for a while, we finally arrived at the large facility.

PART 2

Welcome To Hell

It was May 8, 2013, on the night we arrived. The digital clock on the dashboard from the backseat of the squad car read 8:45 p.m. The sheriff pulled in through the back gate of the old, rundown MCJ (Men's Central Jail) facility. It was said that if you could survive there you could survive any prison, anywhere. It is located in East Los Angeles.

I noticed an unseasonably cold breeze as I peered from the backseat, staring into the starry night sky. I took one long, deep breath before the engine stopped, not knowing when I'd have this picturesque moment again. As the sheriff turned the engine off, his partner came around to the back to let us out, motioning to the tower guards to close the massive gates behind us. Getting out of the car, I lost my balance and tripped as I stepped out. The chronic pain was back. I was still feeling heavily drugged and disoriented from the meds that had been given to me at the psychiatric ward. This was still one big, ongoing nightmare.

'A blur,' I thought as the tall, older deputy helped me regain my footing. He then led me to the inmate line with the other new arrivals. This was another one of the worst days of my life, the first being the night I'd tried to commit suicide. That night was undoubtedly the worst one I could have ever imagined. The events were still fresh in my mind as I stood there in the freezing cold wearing just a summer shirt, bed slippers, and light sweats.

It crossed my mind that I was wearing the same blood-stained clothes I'd had on that night. For some morbid reason, it was a reminder that I wished I had succeeded in what had now become my official failed attempt. The sad thing was nobody here cared. I was just another new inmate, along with the others. It was just another routine inmate-processing day for the sheriffs who were leading us into hell that evening.

"God, please help this broken spirit," I prayed before walking into the massive structure.

"I want you to follow the blue line when you get inside, and follow it all the way down to the end of the hall!" instructed the sheriff in a drill-sergeant tone. "Keep your shoulders off the walls and I want NO talking!"

These, unfortunately, were the words that greeted me my first time in jail. The new inmate arrivals at the MCJ were led in through the back of the large facility. They took off our cuffs and merged us with other inmates from squad cars and buses who were also just arriving. There were enormous, intimidating fences surrounding the building, with layer upon layer of barbed wire on top. Staying on the blue line, we walked down an old, dingy, and seemingly never-ending hall.

On each side of it were rows of holding tanks as far down as the dim lighting would allow you to see. They were rundown and filthy, as though they hadn't been cleaned or maintained in years. They were filled to the brim with gang members, all separated by gang affiliation. There were Crips separated from Bloods,

Latino gangs, and lower-level offenders, who were separated from them as well. There were the Aryan Nation skinheads. Gang inmates in the tanks were flashing gang signs to fellow members and rival gang members in the line. Some of the gang inmates in the line, who were bald, had visible gashes in the back of their heads from previous fights and altercations. Most gang members of all races had tattoos everywhere. It was sad to see that some were disfigured, with teeth missing, caved-in skulls, as well as visible stab and gunshot wounds.

It looked like a fresh war zone in Afghanistan. The system probably saw them all as incorrigible misfits. For some reason, I saw more than that, and I felt for them. This had to be hard on their loved ones. No one is born this way. It felt as if society had bunched them all together and given up on them. I was a new edition to the disturbing images I was witnessing.

Parts of the line were moving slower than others. This was mostly the older gang inmates who had permanent limps from gunshots wounds and years of gang banging. It was sad. I had no understanding of what it all meant, other than what I'd seen on TV. Meanwhile, the guards were beginning to walk up and down the line to make sure we didn't stop or slow down, and that the ones who were limping from gunshot wounds weren't holding us up.

It was so crowded. Every inch of space in the holding tanks was filled with inmates in wait of a bunk. It just didn't seem right that some were lying on hard, filthy concrete floors under benches without blankets. It looked like they were freezing. Some lay there shivering, while others were pacing the floor, yelling out expletives to the guards to let them use the phones so they could call their attorneys. They all looked weary and worn, probably from years of returning to this place as if it were a revolving door.

The rate of recidivism (inmates who return) was high here, another inmate told me. These inmates had already been processed in Reception (where we were headed) and were now waiting—some for days—to be housed in the over-crowded jail population. L.A. has the largest jail population in the U.S. I have always suffered from social anxieties, and this was beyond overwhelming and frightening. As I tried to adjust to this new, dangerous environment, a vexatious feeling came over me. In my head, I kept praying to God, *'Please deliver me from this nightmare.'*

I was exhausted when we finally reached the Reception area. *'So, this is where it all happens,'* I thought. As a somber moment came over me, something was telling me this was all just a bad dream and I would be released soon. I didn't know the procedure for processing an inmate, but I was about to find out soon enough. *'This all has to be some kind of a mistake.'*

All I knew was that the sheriff had called it 'false imprisonment' when they'd arrested me back at the hospital's psychiatric ward. It sounded very serious, but I was yet to find out just how serious those words associated with the accusations really were. We were now being led to a bench amongst the plethora that filled every inch of the spacious and rundown room.

Every which way you turned there were sheriffs. It had the look of an Eighties crime-suspense TV drama.

I was led to a bench with two long chains running through it, and shackled to a row of inmates sitting shoulder-to-shoulder, one attached to our wrist and the other to our ankles. From the grimaces on some of their faces, it appeared they had been sitting there for days, along with a room full of others, all waiting to be processed. The sad part about it was that there was only one doctor to psychologically evaluate all of us, and it would take days of waiting at this rate. I was surrounded by cross-dressing male prostitutes with lipstick and flamboyant wigs on. There were drug dealers on the phone with their attorneys, gang bangers, pimps, attempted suicides—you name it. You didn't have to search far in here to find it.

I couldn't believe my eyes as new inmates kept flooding in by the minute. Some came in with gunshot wounds and others with stabbings. *'How did we all wind up in a place like this?'* I wondered how many of them were spiritual. That was the bigger question yet. No matter how much society judged all of us, we were still God's children. Whether everyone here was spiritual or not, it was still real. *'Why was I trying to commit suicide if I believed in God?'* My spirit was weary. I was tired of trying to figure it out. That incident will haunt me for the rest of my days on this earth.

"Jackson! Next for the doctor!" came the voice of a nurse calling out the next inmate for evaluation. For the next day-and-a-half of sitting in the same position, shackled by ankle and wrist, I heard every name called but mine. I waited impatiently. Finally, my name came ringing over the room's loudspeaker. "Palmer! Next for the doctor!"

I could barely raise my hand. I was so weak from not eating, and both my wrist and throat burned from where I had slashed them.

"You Palmer?" he asked as the nurse pointed me out to the sheriff to come over to release me from the cuffs and chains.

I could barely stand as the sheriff walked alongside me, helping me stand, then following me over to the doctor's room. There was so much confusion. Nurses ran every which way. Deputies walking past with new inmates. It took me a minute just to walk through it all. I stepped into the doctor's office and he motioned for me to sit down in the chair across from him as he talked on the phone. He looked unkempt and worn down from his job. He soon finished his call.

"Are you Robert D. Palmer?" he asked in an East Indian accent. He adjusted his reading glasses to read the charges against me. "These are pretty serious charges," he said with a strong accent, leaning in closer from across the cluttered desk. He showed me the paper with the charges. "Did you do all this?" he asked.

"Do all of what?" I responded.

He told me he wasn't sure what false imprisonment was. "Do you still feel suicidal?" he said, his voice filled with concern.

I told him no. He then ordered the nurse to bring in an electric blood pressure machine. The first one immediately cut off when she connected it to my arm. She went and got another one, and it did the same thing. She said it had never done that before. Then the lights overhead began to flicker. I was used to it, but I'm quite sure they weren't.

"Okay, that will be all I need. Thank you, Mr. Palmer," he said as the sheriff waiting by the door motioned for me to follow him back into the Reception area. "Wait over here," he said, motioning for me to stand by the wall next to a line of other inmates. I was now waiting for them to tell me how the doctor would decide my fate in this war zone.

SUICIDE WATCH

The doctor in the Reception area finally concluded his evaluation (after I had waited a day-and-a-half on a bench, chained shoulder-to-shoulder, ankle-to-ankle to a long row of other inmates). I was to be placed on suicide watch for the next seventy-two hours, or until further notice. I was led down the hall, again chained to a long line of inmates. They took us to a room where we had a shower and were sprayed for lice. Then we were given a long blue one-piece, short-sleeved padded jacket that closed with Velcro. This was also to keep us from using our clothing as makeshift nooses to hang ourselves with. An angry despair came over me as we headed toward the last few feet that curved down to the long hall that housed the suicide-watch pod.

"How many times have you been here?" I asked the disheveled-looking inmate in front of me.

"Shut up! Now!" came the loud and brash orders of a guard. "There'll be no talking in my line. You got that, inmate?" The man stood in front of my face, shouting out the order. He looked like an ex-Marine.

"If anyone in line feels like killing himself or anyone else, you should let one of us know immediately," came the cold and insensitive remark from one of the other guards. He could sense that most in the line were clearly mentally ill and unstable. This was probably why we had been denied bail for release, or anything else for that matter, until further evaluation. Most of the inmates in line, including myself, had visible, fresh suicide attempts on their bodies. Some looked like they had made multiple failed attempts. It resembled a triage in an ER. There was gauze falling off one inmate who had ripped it off, exposing fresh wounds made, perhaps, in the hope of bleeding to death.

We all shared one thing in common: we had no desire to live. We were the new arrivals, entering the land of hopelessness, the wastebasket of society. We were now the new inductees into its infamous 'Hall of Shame'. I'd seen this suicide-watch pod before on TV documentaries, but had never expected its cold grimness to be a part of my reality. I said a short prayer before we arrived. I asked God for strength to meet the unknown.

After a short walk, we arrived at the suicide-watch pod. The pod resembled something from a sci-fi movie. It was very high-tech, sterile, and fairly new. There were rows of them. It was in a pod atmosphere with two open floors of inmate cells. Spyder tables were in the day area. It was overlooked by an impressive, fully automated control room with one-way, smoked-out glass windows. There was a sign that read 'Suicide Watch'.

As we walked up to the door, you could hear multiple clicking sounds of handcuffs being removed, and inmates being led to their cells on the two open floors. Some were without confrontation; others had to be restrained and held down by several guards at a time. The guards were in full combat regalia, some with clear-plastic shields, Tasers, and batons. Some of the inmates were spitting on them, while others smeared feces all over the windows from their cells. Some were screaming at the top of their lungs, exposing their wounds, and letting the blood run in hopes that, maybe if one was an AIDS carrier, he would pass it on to a guard or an inmate.

I couldn't believe what I was seeing. The only problem for some of us was that there weren't enough cells due to overcrowding. The remaining inmates—myself included—were individually chained by the wrist in a supine position. Our wrists were in the air above our heads for the entire time under separate Spyder tables in the dayroom without a break for what seemed days. This gave some of us a birds-eye view of the entire pod.

Later that night, I could hear inmates howling like wild animals caught in traps. Some were banging their heads against the walls. This went on the entire time I was on suicide watch. It never seemed to let up for a minute. It definitely worked on your psyche. It was sad and disturbing. Watching guards enter cells and have to wrestle down certain unruly inmates was hard for me to bear. I just lay there and recited prayers I remembered from the Bible, asking God to deliver each and every one of our spirits from that wretched place. Prayers for the lost, as I was myself. Prayers of strength to overcome the despair and loneliness that had overcome my spirit each minute that passed. "God, please don't let me lose this crushing battle."

I'd now lost all sense of time. I could no longer feel emotions. I just lay there, quiet and dazed, my arm hanging by a blood-stained cuff from a failed suicide attempt. Every so often a guard would walk by to make sure we weren't trying to kill ourselves again.

After lying there for a day-and-a-half, a guard I thought was making his typical rounds came over to me, bent down, and took the dried-blood-stained cuffs off my wrist from the table seat. *'Thank God,'* I thought. *'They don't have credible evidence against me and are finally setting me free. God has heard my prayers after all.'*

"Let me see your wristband. You Palmer?" he asked with some compassion as he removed the cuff.

I was so weak from self-induced starvation and lying in that position for so long that I barely had the strength to answer. I mustered up just enough strength to respond. "Yes, I am."

"Wrap up your roll and get in that line over there," he instructed.

I was finally getting out of this hellhole. I was so weak that another inmate came over to help me get into the line.

"Single file. Line it up in a single file. Now!" came the command from the sergeant.

We made our way toward the door. I turned around one last time to get a final glimpse of hell as we made our way down the hall, passing several other pods, and onto an elevator. When it opened, that's when I noticed...

In The Lion's Den, Part 1

We had passed by the Prisoner Release line. I had thought I was going to be released. What happened was confusing. I was being transferred from the Suicide Watch floor to the floor where they housed 'the Yellows'. It was the mental facility part of the jail, where historically some of the most notorious psychopaths, sociopaths, and criminally-insane inmates were housed while awaiting trial. They were called Yellows because of the yellow tops worn to distinguish them from the other inmates. We were part of a large group of inmates that day who were being transported by a group of ten heavily-armed guards to the floor where the Yellows' pod was located.

"Follow the blue line, single file, and stay against the wall at all times," a guard yelled out.

I still had it in my mind that I was being released at any minute. How could they hold me for more than the seventy-two-hour mental evaluation? "This is just all too surreal," I kept telling myself, unaware that the real nightmare was just beginning. This was how oblivious I was to how the penal system here worked and where I was being transferred—all based on an allegation. An allegation had put me there and, in time, would profoundly alter the spiritual course of my life to this very day.

"I want all men to line up single file, get fully undressed, grab yourselves a yellow, and get dressed. Line up single file and grab yourself a roll-up as you walk by me!" instructed the head guard.

A roll-up is a blanket that includes one sheet, underwear, toiletries, a toothbrush, toothpaste, and a roll of toilet paper with a bar of soap wedged between it. These were the allotted weekly rations, and if you ran out you were tough out of luck. The toothpaste tasted like cardboard. The blanket was so lightweight you froze most of the time. The temperature in the dorms and cellblock was usually kept brutally cold. This, I was told, was to keep the staph infections down to a minimum. Judging by the number of inmates who contracted it, the problem was not contained very well. It was at that moment that an inmate came over to inform me I was on the wrong bunk.

"You aren't in the dorm area. You're in a two-man cellblock!" he shouted, pointing over across the dorm to cellblock 2.

Something didn't feel right after he yelled out, judging by the swarm of inmates who were now following us over to it. We could now hear a loud ruckus emanating from within the cell walls, which was impossible to see because the inmate who occupied it had covered all the windows with newspaper. All I could hear was this bombastic, heavy voice, yelling out every expletive known to man. He was yelling how no one was ever coming in again, and if anyone came in now, it would be pretty bad for them. I froze in sheer terror. Were they actually going to put me in there with him?

The door to cellblock 2A clicked open with a loud, clunking thud. It was now unlocked. A momentary silence fell over the entire dorm. Then, over the loudspeaker came the blaring of the guard commanding me to enter the cell. "Palmer! Enter cellblock 2A!!"

I feared for my life! Whoever was on the other side of that door slammed it back shut. "Aww, come on, Sam. Let this one in," came the plea from a high-powered, black Crip gang member. Next came the sound from inside of someone's body ramming the cell door at full impact, shaking the cell walls. I knew there was no way in hell I was going into that cell without a sheriff guard or an inmate escort, especially knowing that whoever was on the other side of that door was waiting to rip me apart.

After what seemed like an hour of useless coercion, the door finally flew open. To my dismay, standing and blocking the cell entrance was this deranged-looking, six-foot-six white inmate who was as big as Shrek. He appeared to be in his late twenties.

"Let 'em in, Sam!" pleaded a Southsider, a Latino gang member.

"I told you ain't nobody crossing this line as long as I'm breathing! You got that?" he shouted back.

I stood there and stared in disbelief at his size in proportion to the cell. I tried convincing one of the other inmates to change my cell. My pleas fell on deaf ears. It was at that moment of God's saving grace that a guard saw the commotion, came over, ordered the inmates to disperse, and for Sam to let me into the cell or else he would lockdown the entire floor. This did nothing but agitate him further; when the guard left, I would be the unlucky recipient stuck in the cell with him.

With reluctance and a cold, blank stare on his face, he slowly stepped aside to let me in. I walked in cautiously, knowing not to take my eyes off him, not even for a moment, or else it could turn fatal. I surveyed the landscape of the tight quarters. It was truly depressing: the cell conditions were dilapidated, rundown, and deplorable. It was complete squalor. There was one stack of rusted metal bunks in a cell that was about six-by-ten feet. There also was a small metal table and a stainless-steel sink and toilet. The basic essentials.

The lower bunk I assumed was mine. I could feel the intensity from his eyes again beaming on me. As I made up my bunk, I felt a sense of trepidation. Not a word was spoken between us. I wasn't sure how to initiate the conversation, especially when there was an uncomfortable silence unlike anything I'd ever experienced before. I had never been to jail in my entire life! My heart thumped through my chest like a jackhammer pounding through concrete pavement.

In those next few minutes, all I could hear spinning in my head was, *'I'm actually here in this hellhole!'* It just didn't compute, and to make matters worse, when I was arrested, no one handed me a Survival Guide or a handbook on 'how to survive being locked in a cell with a psychopath'. All I had was God on my side, and my spirit was about to be tested in ways I'd ever encountered.

As night fell over us, he walked around the cell, slamming things into the wall. I tried my best to hide my fear, but it was obvious to every inmate that this was my first time around the block. This was their world. They could smell fear in you a mile away. I made up my mind that the only way I was going to survive this nightmare was to stay awake, keep my eyes on him, and pray to God throughout it. I sat in a lotus position with my back to the wall, propping myself up to keep from falling asleep.

In jail, hours seem to pass like days. You feel every solitary minute of it. Hours had now passed. He still hadn't taken his eyes off me, nor had a word been spoken between us. It was at that moment I noticed he had a bird's quill in his hand and was sharpening it on the cement floor. Out of nowhere, he blurted out, "That's why they got me here in the Yellows," in a monotone voice. "They think I'm crazy or deranged or something, simply because I split my best friend's head open with the butt of a gun! I tried to kill him. He stole something precious from me. He deserved it! He was lucky I didn't shoot him with it," he told me as he continued to stare at me.

I could still hear the scraping sound, but not for a minute was I going to take my eyes off him yet. We sat there in those positions for the remainder of the night. There was no way I was going to sleep. I made it through the night, and he finally gave up, climbed up on his bunk, and went to sleep. But tomorrow was another day.

"Chow! Time for chow!" came the sound over the loudspeakers. The smell of the food was nauseating. An inmate came to the door and called Sam as he got up and disappeared into the dorm to eat. "Whew!" I was relieved, if only for the moment. Here I was, on a twenty-four-hour/seven-days-a-week lockdown. *'How long will I be stuck in this horrid place with this inmate? Will I survive here? Is God trying to reveal something to me here?'* But there were no answers to my questions. Just silence.

"God, why did You keep me alive? Was it to punish me for attempting to kill myself? I need answers and I need them now! I am all alone here."

I stayed in the cell for most of the day. Sam stayed out in the dorm until the loudspeaker announcement: "All inmates, you have five minutes to lock it down!' echoed the guard. "Get in your cells and lock it down. Get ready for night count!"

The dorm inmate rep was now calling out the same words behind him. "You heard him. Lock it down, guys, so the sheriff will turn the TV back on!"

You could now hear the metallic sound of cell doors slamming one by one, bringing the night to a close. It was just him and me again in a dark, cold cell. How would it play out this time?

IN THE LION'S DEN, PART 2

From the way I saw it, it played out in one word, and that word was F-E-A-R. I was starting to learn that, in jail, there's usually only one way for most things in a high-level-security, mental ward pod to play out, and that's through pure, unadulterated FEAR

It was the ultimate fear: Sam now back in the cell, staring me down again, continuing to sharpen the bird quill on the cement floor. He was now breathing heavily, panting like a rabid animal in the wild, when the sound of guards' feet coming for night count brought a momentary distraction of relief. It drew his attention away from me.

Fear is that one emotion that can strangle all the other senses inside you in a single second. It affects all judgment. It can affect your psyche. It is the darkest of all emotions known to man.

I now was being held firm within its clutches and experiencing a panic/anxiety attack. The chronic joint pain was back. I was having trouble breathing and was getting weaker from the self-imposed suicidal-induced starvation, which was now starting to cause delirium. As the guard's voice commanded us to stand up, approach the cell door window, and show him our wristband name and numbers, I could barely stand and was too weak to respond. The blaring sound of his voice penetrated my eardrum like the horn of a diesel.

As the guards resumed their night count through the pod, Sam paced the floor without uttering a word. Suddenly he walked past me and jumped up onto his bunk. He was getting stranger and more agitated by the moment, I could tell. I trusted him even less now. Even though his bunk was above me and I couldn't see him, I could still feel the tension in the room as if he were planning his moment of attack soon, and it was all about to come to a head. Maybe this was my chance to finally close my weary eyes. Or, maybe not. Maybe that's what he was waiting for me to do. Earlier, he'd had that sly, piercing look in his eyes like he knew I would soon run out of strength and answers, and I was bound to get caught slipping if I fell asleep. The lost and rundown within me was mounting exponentially as I lay waiting and wondering when his moment of attack would come.

The thing to do was not fall asleep again, at any cost. Stay awake by any means necessary. But I was so exhausted, I kept losing sense of my surroundings and time. I somehow kept thinking I was at home in my apartment and this was all a delusion. But it wasn't. It was real—so real that I had to regain my senses quickly. Every few minutes, I would fall back to let my head bump the wall just to stay awake. Then I squeezed the slashed areas of my wrist in hopes that the intense pain would also keep me awake. It was excruciating. How much longer could I hold out? Only time would tell. All of this was starting to take a toll on me.

I desperately needed God. I needed Him to help me through this fear that had me in its grips. Those were the prayers going through my mind. Here I was, never having been to jail, now fighting to keep my sanity within mindsight, despite what was happening in our cell. I was in a cell with a psychopath. Would praying help? I wasn't sure. If it did, then why was I here? I had a bone to pick with God.

An hour had passed and I could hear the guards preparing to make their second nighttime hourly rounds. *'Finally!'* I thought, as the lights were brought up from dimly-lit to brighter than a department store. I asked him why they made so many rounds at night. "To make sure you aren't dead," was his answer.

When he left, Sam jumped down from his bunk and furiously paced the floor, mumbling to himself. It sounded morbid, strange, and indecipherable. It was almost as if they had thwarted his plan. He sat down in front of me and said, "I can tell by looking into people's eyes if they're getting ready to lie to me." I didn't know where that had just come from, but he kept repeating it as his breathing got heavier.

'What was wrong with him?' I wondered. *'Why does he have so much anger and rage inside him?'*

When I came in he'd told them he wanted to be alone. Maybe he was afraid of what he was capable of doing to an inmate in his cell. After all, he was a predator, that was clear, and whoever was in there with him was his prey. He was evil personified. He could kill me quickly and no one would care. He would probably be doing me a favor, except I didn't want to die by the brutal shanking of a bird quill in my neck. It was too gruesome to think about. This went on throughout the rest of the night, hour after hour, between the guards' shifts into the early morning. Maybe he was trying to wear me down by some psychological game. Finally, the early call out came for breakfast.

"Wake it up for chow! It's chow time!"

Whew! I exhaled in relief. I had now made it through another night. I was now into day eight of my suicide-by-starvation attempt. I couldn't hold out much longer at this level.

"God, since you won't hear my plea, please let me hurry up and die peacefully. I don't want to deal with any more of this agony."

Without saying a word, he sat down in front of me and smiled for the first time since I'd arrived. "You gonna eat breakfast?" he asked. I was stunned. That was all he said, then he disappeared out into the dorm. I thought, 'What just happened?' This was just too much. I needed to calm my nerves, so I decided to meditate. 'Maybe I just need to talk to Sam.' I thought I was delusional at that moment. This out-of-control inmate probably wanted nothing more than to stick me in the neck.

Later that day when Sam came in, he seemed to be in a better mood, for some reason. He was less agitated. What had touched his spirit? Where was all that rage he'd had since I first met him? It was very confusing. I was still reluctant to talk to him, but I thought, 'What do I have to lose?' I told Sam I had something to talk to him about, knowing I was still a stranger to him. He responded with hesitation then agreed to hear me. He reminded me again of his ability to tell whether someone was lying to him, and he didn't know what he was capable of if they did. After he gave me that warning, I hesitated.

He sat on the small stool attached to the metal table next to it. He looked at me with that blank, dark stare. I knew I had to choose carefully the next words that came from my mouth. *'God, please touch this inmate.'* I first asked him if he believed in God.

"No; that's for people who are weak," he said with a sarcastic look.

"Well, He believes in you," I told him. "He wants me to tell you about your childhood, how you were abandoned several times as a child by your parents."

"Wow! You couldn't have known that!" he yelled out. "No way you could've known that! That's impossible!"

I just knew I'd pissed him off. After that, he stared at me for a few minutes before he responded. I just knew he was going to shank me. He began to tell me how his dad had left them when he was four. When he was five, his mother was in another room of the house and he'd called out to her, but she didn't answer. He went into the room and saw her lying there dead. He said he'd felt abandoned by both of them. He then went to stay with his grandmother. He lived with her for a few years. One day, he went outside to play, and when he came back in, she was lying on the floor dead.

"Oh my God!" I said in shock. *'What a horrible story,'* I thought.

He went on to tell me that he totally shut down at this point and felt the ultimate abandonment. That's when he said the violence started.

Our talk went on for a while when, suddenly, he burst into tears and his head just dropped in my lap. I didn't know what to do. I had never witnessed such a strong response. He said there was no way I could have known that. I put my hands on his head and shoulders and held him as if he were my own son. His story was so gut-wrenching that my tears began to flow. I couldn't believe what was happening, but it was real.

'Could this be my calling? Is God trying to tell me something?'

Sam raised his head and said something had moved inside him. He said no one had ever cried for him since he was a kid. It reminded him of when he was younger. He said what I somehow knew had really gotten to him.

"How long have you been doing this?" he asked.

I told him I'd just started with him. He was genuinely shocked. He'd never had God in his life.

"It was God, not me, Who touched you," I told him.

Maybe Sam just needed someone to care about him and look beneath that hard veneer he displayed in the dorm. Maybe he'd been so neglected as a child it had shaped his personality into this dark soul he'd portrayed. Maybe his anger was his armor and the only way he knew of protecting the child inside him. He was wiping the tears so the other inmates wouldn't see as he stood up and began to pace the floor in disbelief. I could tell he wasn't used to showing his feelings around anyone except his grandma, and I wasn't used to the response he'd shown as well. He soon disappeared into the dorm with the other inmates.

I still couldn't get over his reaction. I thought about how my suicide-by-starvation plan had been going on for almost eight days. At that point, for some undefinable reason, I'd felt it pointless to continue with it any longer, especially after what had just happened with Sam. With all the remaining energy I could muster, I stood there in the cell by myself. I was in my boxers and in shock as I stared at my emaciated frame through the reflection of the dingy, soot-smeared window. Through it, I could faintly make out that my stubbly, grey beard had noticeably filled in and I looked detestably older. By this time I was starting to take on the transient jail and starvation look.

Later that night, when Sam returned to the cell, he actually helped me out of bed and walked me to the food line. He commented on what had happened earlier. His words were, "Can I start calling you Preach?" I just laughed. "No, really?" he kept saying. He also commented on how small I was and said he was happy I was eating again. We stood there and got more acquainted as he held me up while we waited for chow. He shared with me again about his violent past. I couldn't believe what I was hearing.

We got back to the cell with our trays and began exchanging food. I gave him most of mine because it looked disgusting and I knew I had to go slow. I sat at the small table by the bunk and thought about how he had been institutionalized from coming in and out so much that he probably no longer noticed how bad it really was. That was sad.

I went to bed that night thinking about the events of the day and how awesome God was. Here I was, in a strange place with violence all around me, yet there was a calm I was starting to feel from Him. *'No one would believe me if I told them this story,'* I thought as I lay there and prayed for thanks and deliverance from this dreadful, inhumane place.

I grabbed the thin blanket, pulled it up over me to break the frigid-cold air streaming in from the vent, curled up tightly in it, and soon nodded off to sleep. I knew it would be count-time soon; I always slept light until the last count of the evening. Before Sam went to bed that night he asked me to show him how to pray. I did and he said he would try to remember to do it at night.

A few days later, as I stood waiting to be transferred, Sam walked up and hugged me from behind. "Preach, yeah, that should be your name. Promise me you'll keep it?"

I laughed and promised him. I left the dorm, not knowing where they were placing me next. I was living minute-by-minute, but I now knew God was with me, and in knowing that, it brought me comfort.

A VISIT FROM ANGELS

Weeks had now passed and there hadn't been a word from my family. I imagined by now they knew something was wrong, especially as I didn't send out cards for Mother's Day weeks previously. That was something I always did. I was worried they wouldn't have a way to reach me, until one day the loud voice spoke through the intercom: "Palmer! You've got a visitor! Head to the door!" I'd just gotten a pass from the sheriff, telling me the chaplain wanted to see me. I got dressed and came to the front of the pod. The sheriff checked my wristband, then handed me the pass.

I went over to the table where the chaplain was and sat down. He introduced himself as Charles. He was middle-aged and Latino. He proceeded to tell me that my daughter China had tried to reach me. *'Finally, someone from my family has found me,'* I thought. That was comforting. He gave me her number and told me to call her right away. I took it and put it in my pocket. I thanked him as I got up to leave. *'Thank God for chaplains,'* I thought as I walked back to the pod.

When I got back I immediately went to the telephones. The phones were segregated, so I had to use the black ones. I didn't reach her the first time I called, and I was anxious and nervous. It felt awkward calling her from a jail phone. I wasn't quite used to it yet. I tried her an hour later and finally she answered.

"Oh my God, Dad!!" she cried out. It had to have been hard on her. I tried to keep her spirits up. I asked her if she had called any other of my family members. She said she didn't have anyone's number. I told her the story of how I'd wound up incarcerated. Naturally, she was shocked, especially about the suicide part. She started crying again. She asked me when my court date was.

"It's in twenty days. Let's just hope when I go that this thing will all be over, and the judge will let me get out of here,' I said, trying to sound reassuring.

She asked what I was going to do about my apartment and possessions. I told her I wasn't sure. It was hard conversing with inmates listening in on your every word.

"Do you want Emmett and me to come out to California and put your things in storage?"

I told her yes; I didn't have any other options. I was truly grateful, knowing she would have to take time away from her job and the children. She said they would catch the next flight out and immediately take care of it. I was relieved. She was extremely reliable. I went back to my bunk excited. I hadn't seen my daughter in years—we'd only communicated by cell—but I wasn't sure I wanted her to see me like this under these conditions.

I lay there and stared at the ceiling, thinking about everything that had transpired in the last few months. It was overwhelming. The call came out for chow. I was excited because it temporarily took my mind off things. Even if only for a short time, it was still worth it.

A couple of days passed and I was excited about this particular one. Today, I was going to see my baby, my daughter China. I had butterflies. I had missed her so much. I waited impatiently for my name to be called. To get out of this hellhole for a few minutes was worth it. Finally, around midday, the sound of my name called over the loudspeaker brought chills to my arms. I quickly jumped down from my bunk and got ready. I went up to the pod door and showed the guard my wristband. "You, Palmer?" I answered, "Yes, sir."

He stepped aside and let me out the door. He pointed toward the direction of the visiting section. Slowly, I walked over and sat in one of the assigned cubicles. I was nervous. I sat there for a few minutes and the prettiest twenty-eight-year-old girl in the world, my daughter, sat down in front of the glass between us. We both cried. This wasn't the way I wanted her to see me. I was unshaven and scraggly looking, but I am what I am, and I had to face that truth—I was in jail. There was nothing glamorous about it in the least. We put our hands to the glass in a gesture of touching each other. There wasn't much time. We were only allotted fifteen minutes, so we tried to make the best of it. She gave me a book to sign my power of attorney over to her so she could handle my affairs.

I was so proud of her. She'd stepped up to the plate for her dad. I was so grateful. Your kids will always be your babies no matter what age they are, I thought. China has two beautiful daughters with Emmett, her Liberian fiancé. She asked what I wanted to do about my apartment. I told her I wasn't sure how long I would be in jail. She said they would clear it out and put everything in storage for me. I was thankful to God that He had given me such a wonderful daughter and her fiancé, as well as the rest of my children. She said she would notify the rest of the family and tell them what had happened.

Our fifteen minutes went fast, but we got to say what was important. It was still bittersweet, me seeing her and her having to leave so quickly. She got up to leave and threw me a kiss as she walked out of sight. I went back to my pod. I was very proud of her. I was feeling melancholy as I arrived back at my bunk. Thoughts of why I was incarcerated were getting the best of me. I had been in jail for over a month now. I just wanted the day to hurry up and end, but not before I thanked God for such a loving and caring daughter and son-in-law-to-be. I slept well that night.

An Exchange For A Miracle

My court date had finally come. It felt like an entire year had passed. In jail, you feel every single minute that passes, and it can wear you down fast if you don't quickly develop a coping mechanism for it. Now I see why some inmates were walking around in almost catatonic states. I was finally going to get my chance to prove my innocence.

Unfortunately, when I took the long bus ride across town, it was for nothing. My attorney was out of town, so the judge postponed it for another thirty days. I couldn't believe I would have to spend another minute in that wretched place. The accusations were false, and I needed my chance in court to prove it. I already had been there thirty days too long, and it was beginning to wear me down even more. I wasn't cut out for incarceration.

When I got back to my cell, I had to try to make sense of it all. The permeating stench of it from all the years of built-up rust and mildew. The worn mattress, and my chronic joint pain, which was now relentless. All of these things only exacerbated my depression even more. I had hit the wall of life, and I couldn't push this body and spirit any further. When you've prayed for something for so many years and there are times when you've just given up, what do you do? You wonder if God has heard your prayers.

I sat there with all remaining hope now gone. God knew I couldn't get any lower than this. In that moment, it had become so excruciating that I banged my arm into the wall just to deflect the pain from it. In jail they won't give you anything stronger than ibuprofen, which doesn't help. I was now out on a raft in the middle of the sea of uncertainty. I needed stronger meds.

"I saw how You used me and what You did back there with Sam, how he gave me this nickname, Preach. But what do I do with it from here?"

I picked up the Bible from the table and thumbed through it. I read a few passages, put it down, then closed my eyes to pray.

"Dear Father God. I'm at the end of this rope. All my faith has been challenged these last twenty years. I don't know what this all means. But what I do know is I need You unlike any time I ever have in my life! Please give me a sign of what I should do at this point. Please take this pain off me forever, and I promise to minister to the inmates in here. I don't know how to preach, but please give me a pain-free body to do it with."

I meditated well into the late hours of that night, with a feeling in my spirit unlike anything I'd known before. Had He heard me?

I can't explain what happened that evening. Something was definitely different. I now felt the spirit of God was going to guide me. For the first time in my spiritual life I was willing to totally surrender to Him. I had nothing to lose. There was a lot of work somebody could do in here. I had nothing else to do every day; maybe this was the very reason I was here. Maybe this place was my house of surrender. I could make good use of my time there, unlike on the outside.

I couldn't believe how excited I was. God was clearing a path in His own mysterious way for me to develop an intimate relationship with Him unlike any I'd experienced before. But how would I start? I wasn't a preacher. I'd never done a Bible study or prayer and worship for anyone in my life. What made me think I could do it? Then I remembered Jesus said, "All you have to do is ask and the Holy Spirit will come."

I felt that a cloud had been lifted. For the rest of that day, I walked around the jail pod in a daze. A gang member came over to me and said he'd seen me intensely meditating that night. "Hey, OG. What's your name?"

I thought about it for a minute, then remembered Sam had called me Preach. "My name's Robert, but they call me Preach."

"Okay, Preach, you think you can show me how to do that?"

I was taken aback by his request. "Sure, I can show you."

So, I did. More inmates started crowding around, having me show them as well. What was happening?

When I came back to my bunk to meditate, I suddenly noticed I hadn't had any pain all day. That was very unusual because the pain the previous evening was some of the worst I'd experienced in some time. Now it was suddenly gone? I knew it was too early to get excited, but I couldn't help it. I just thought, give it a few hours and it has to come back.

It was now going into the late hours of the night and still no pain. Had God removed it from me? I hadn't gone pain-free this long in over twenty years. And if so, for how long? I got in a lotus position and started to meditate. I asked Him, "Is this really happening? Is this a miracle You have given me in exchange for ministering to the inmates? This is something I've prayed to You for many years to take away; why now? Back when I died and just before You brought me back to life, where did I go? Was that a glimpse of heaven You showed me? I believe for the first time since that night that maybe this was the reason You didn't let me stay there. After all of those years, maybe Your reason for bringing me back was to come here and minister to these inmates? Maybe You removed all of my pain to allow me to do it. I now believe I'm sure of it, to share with the inmates that I'm a walking miracle of hope for them, and even myself. And for that, I am forever grateful to You."

Tears of joy streamed down my face. I was overtaken with deep gratitude. I was beginning to see that what I'd endured for so many years had brought me to this moment of truth. Jesus said, "If any of you wants to be My follower, you must give up your own way, take up your cross, and follow Me. If you try to hang onto your life, you will lose it. But if you give up your life for My sake, you will save it. And what do you benefit if you gain the whole world but lose your own soul?"

This was uncharted territory, but if I was going to preach, there could be 'no more fear.'

PRAYERS FOR A CUTTER

I had now been incarcerated in the L.A. County Jail for three months. By the psychiatric evaluation I'd just taken again, they'd determined I was neither crazy nor deemed a threat to myself or suicidal. So, for the depression, they were now transferring me to another part of the mental ward—the infamous 'Twin Towers', the largest mental facility in the world. Unfortunately, it happens to be in a jail. It houses thousands of the mentally ill in a heavily-guarded, lockdown atmosphere. It ranges from the low-level mentally ill to the criminally insane. From dangerous psychopaths and sociopaths to psychotic murderers—you name it, they have it there. Because of that, I found myself surrounded by some of the most mentally afflicted I'd ever heard or read about in my life. It was truly a sobering sight to witness.

My state-of-mind had improved considerably, and I was taking a low-dose medication for the first time to stabilize the mood swings brought on by the depression. I felt it was working. What was helping the most was the serenity brought on by meditation. Through it, I was finally beginning to find the clarity I'd needed and sought for most of my life. Maybe this place represented another life lesson God was still teaching me since I'd been incarcerated. By showing up for others, God was teaching me how to show up for myself. That I meant something special to Him and He wanted to show me just what that 'special something' was.

After getting settled and putting my belongings away in my bunk, I later went out into the jail pod. I found myself trying not to be overly shocked or judgmental at some of the disturbing things I was seeing. Because after all, this was going to be my home—for God only knew how long. I had lunch, then I sat on the end of my bunk in a lotus position and meditated for my usual three-and-a-half hours. It was peaceful. Any worries or doubt seemed to dissipate immediately. This new comforting space that God was providing for me had me believing everything in my life was finally going to be all right, despite where I was and what these conditions represented. He was showing me, "You can be in any situation, but spiritually not of it."

Afterward, an inmate with a wild hairdo, very fair-skinned, who looked to be bi-racial, walked up to me. I was taken aback by the juxtaposition of his nerdiness and the jail surroundings. I introduced myself to him simply as Preach. He said his name was Jeffrey Adams, but they called him Zigzag and that was exactly what the name meant. We had a good laugh… until it went cold in my heart, like I'd just walked outside and was frostbitten in a -25°F blizzard, when I noticed he had more cut marks up both of his arms than a railroad track to Texas. Then, I was hit by a sudden wave of sadness for him.

"Oh, these?" he said.

I had tried not to be so obvious, but he must've detected it.

"It's okay, Preach. I'm just a God-loving, nerdy meth-head, with a degree in biology from Stanford."

Whew! How about that for a combination!

"Oh yeah, and I forgot one: I'm a cutter also."

I just scratched my head and followed him as he went over and grabbed a couple of milks for us. He then walked me over to an empty Spyder table, where we both sat. He had a large, bound Bible, filled with more colored markers than a kid's jumbo crayon box.

"Why do you have so many markers?" I asked.

"Well, when you take a nerd and give him a Bible, I guess this is what you get."

He laughed and told me about his time at Stanford as a biologist, and how just before graduating, he descended into using crystal-meth. He eventually became strung-out and later found himself on the streets of L.A., homeless. He said he was always getting arrested for harassing and scaring someone on the streets for money to buy drugs.

I could see this poor young man was part of a vicious cycle, and because California had shut down all of its mental facilities, the only place left for people like himself was L.A. County's Twin Tower Mental Facility. This place was like a small city. I couldn't believe how massive it was.

We sat there for hours, and as I got to know him better, he would turn out to be one of the smartest and funniest people I'd met in a long time. He had such a beautiful, infectious spirit. He was as knowledgeable as someone who'd just come out of a seminary school, and yet he was in here. It was puzzling and sad to see all of this talent wasting away in this horrid place.

Later that night, Zigzag led the prayer group and Bible study. He would instantly quote Bible passages and knew them inside-out. I was very impressed with his commitment to God's Word. This went on for weeks, until one day he asked me to lead the prayer group and study. I told him he was doing a fine job, and asked why he needed me. He said he'd overheard me at another table doing it, and it would be good if he could take a break once in a while. I agreed and did it that night for him. After that, he pushed me to do it every night. I did, and really enjoyed working with some of the other inmates.

I'd noticed that more cutters were now being transferred to our jail pod. For the most part, they were shy and kept to themselves. Most of the cut marks were visible because in L.A. County Jail long sleeves are forbidden. They were between nineteen and twenty-two years old, and were there on meth charges and suicide attempts. Nobody really bothered them because most of the other inmates in there had enough severe mental problems of their own to deal with.

At times they'd walk by the Spyder table where I was conducting a prayer group with a curious look on their face, but would quickly look away when I noticed them.

"Why don't you come join us?" I asked one who was looking.

Quickly, he ran and disappeared into the crowd of inmates. I thought I'd keep trying, and maybe one day, they would come sit down to join us.

That day didn't take very long to come around. That particular morning when I came to the Spyder table for Bible study, it was filled with most of them. Zigzag had persuaded them to come, and it was a happy sight to see. But, in the back of my mind I was trying to understand why they'd showed up all of a sudden. Each one introduced himself. First, there was Andy, who had bright red hair and freckles. Then, there was Jackson, who had tats and piercings over most of his body and had a slur from so much meth use. There was Benton, who seemed the shyest at the table. Steve, who was black, was at least six-foot-three and towered over everybody at the table. He said he loved playing basketball but had recently tried to commit suicide again. Louis was the last one to introduce himself and said he'd recently made another suicide attempt as well.

I could see they'd all come from different backgrounds, including myself, but what we all had in common was that we'd forgotten what loving ourselves felt like. I read a passage from the Bible about self-love, Philippians 4:13: *I can do all things through Christ who strengthens me.* They were very attentive, and asked me to read more passages to them. Some had a lot of questions about redemption and salvation. I shared with them some great passages in the Bible from Jesus. It had gone well. They said they would all come back in the morning to learn more. Then we all stood and hugged each other, and I said a prayer at the end.

After most had left and the jail pod was shutting down for the night, I had to ask Zigzag how he'd talked them into attending.

"Preach, look at your wrists. Look at your throat. That's how. We see you as one of us, just a spiritual teaching version, that's all." We laughed and hugged each other, and I thanked him.

Heading to my bunk, I couldn't help but be deeply touched by those heartfelt words and to see those brave young men taking small steps to learn about God. Speaking of learning, I was learning so much that I'd never known about life, and a lot of it after being incarcerated. Working with others had become very cathartic. I was seeing that there is still beauty to be found in this life, no matter where you are and how obtuse things may seem at times.

I did my meditation before going to sleep, and when I asked God what was my spiritual takeaway from this night's powerful lesson, He said, "I needed to choose a shepherd that was familiar to them. One who's still healing from being broken and scarred himself. One to teach them the Word, that he's still learning, to lead these precious sheep back to my fold. Now you see why tonight they've come home." I cried myself to sleep after that.

In those next few weeks, we all spent a lot of time together. I taught them how to meditate and get closer to God. Andy and Jackson vowed to try to stop cutting and even attempting suicide. The others said it was going to take some time, but they were open to reading the Bible more and learning how to love themselves. That's when I told them that God is our Potter and sometimes one of His jars falls off the shelf and breaks. He picks it up to mend it, and after it's fixed, the places where it was cracked—the scars—are still visible for others who are broken. This is our reminder of who the Potter is. That's when I showed them the scars on my stomach from the surgery I'd had when I accidentally overdosed years ago, and the fresh ones on my wrists and throat.

"These are some of the same scars some of you have and the ones that others in life might have but only on the inside. But He is a God Who can heal all of us. If we can accept that He is our Potter, it allows us to feel His deep love and compassion for all of us—the hurt and the brokenness. What's even more important is that He needs us to be alive to show others His work. It's become my new purpose to live, and I hope one day it becomes all of yours."

Then I told them, "Seven ways we could find to die will never be greater than one good reason for us all to live."

We were all empowered that evening, and over that last month I'd grown to love these young men as my own. They were proven fighters to me. I'd learned so much from their strength. I knew that would probably be the last night I'd ever see them again in my life, so I had each one present at the table—Jackson, Steve, Andy, Louis, Benton, and, last but not least, Zigzag—to stand up and run his hands over the scars on the arms of each inmate at the table. I wanted each of us to feel the healing at work and the love of our Potter, GOD.

That time did come. Later that night my name was called to roll it up and be at the main door in ten minutes. I'd now done this a few times and knew the goodbyes had to be short. All the guys were waiting at the door when I got there after packing. I was touched. I hugged each one of them and assured them they could do this thing called life. "Just try to remember, when life seems to spin out of control like mine did, know that your Potter loves you because you're special to him. Let Him heal you. There are always professionals out there to help you as well. Don't be afraid or ashamed to reach out to them." They agreed they would.

The loud sound of the metal door clicked and I knew it was time. I walked away from the pod waving at them. Some of their faces were pressed up against the glass, and they were waving like kids at a carnival. I waved back until their faces seemed to get magically smaller, and eventually, were out of sight. It was a very painful moment.

What I was learning from my own suicide attempt and listening to the stories of what those brave young men had shared about theirs was: When those internal voices of despair (like mine and so many others) are crying out, they can get caught like a candle in a headwind and be quickly extinguished before the distress call can even be heard by someone who can help. Then it's too late. Maybe this can result in one attempting suicide.

Below is an excerpt from Zigzag's letter, copied from his original handwritten version.

MR. PALMER,
I JUST WANTED TO THANK YOU FORMALLY WITH THIS LETTER SO THAT YOU WOULD REALLY SENSE THE IMMENSE GRATITUDE I HAVE IN TERMS OF THE INCREASED SPIRITUAL GROWTH I'VE EXPERIENCED FROM SINCE I'VE HAD THE PRIVILEGE IN STUDYING WITH YOU IN FELLOWSHIP.

I WILL PURSUE THIS ENDEAVOR WHICH IS MY WALK WITH CHRIST FOR THE REST-OF-MY-LIFE. YOUR GIFT IS VERY PRACTICAL AND YOUR COMPASSION FOR THE HUMAN CONDITION IS EXTRAORDINARILY SPECIAL. GOD BLESS YOUR LIFE DEAR FRIEND AND MAY GOD CONTINUALLY BLESS YOU IN YOUR STEWARDSHIP IN SERVING THE LIVING GOD. MUCH LOVE AND RESPECT.

IN LOVING FELLOWSHIP,
JEFFREY CURTIS ADAMS JR.

THE BLUES

I woke up feeling drained that day. I was missing my family, but was glad I'd finally gotten in touch with them recently through my wonderful daughter China. I somehow had gotten used to being in the Yellows, despite it being frantic and unpredictably dangerous most of the time. This day was just like any other day; the usual mental inmate having to be cuffed and escorted out by several guards because he'd gone psycho on another inmate. Or, if he'd tried to hang himself in his cell, they'd transfer him back to Suicide Watch.

I constantly prayed for the dorm and their alleged victims on the outside: James, the psychopathic murderer, was facing life in a mental institution for allegedly cutting up his victim. He could be cold and calculating, and had an eerie presence about him. Allen, the paranoid schizophrenic, who'd allegedly killed two men for messing with his girlfriend. Chris, another psychopath, who'd allegedly bashed in his best friend's head (the man was lucky to have survived). Fred, who had every Bible passage he could get tattooed over his entire body, usually stood in the corner praying to the sky. Who knows who he was actually talking to. They wanted to put him in a mental institution as well.

Those were the kinds of inmates I was around every day, and we were in a high-security, twenty-four/seven lockdown unit. Some of those inmates were already sentenced and waiting to be transferred to Patton State Hospital in San Bernardino for the criminally insane. I tried to bring as many as I could to God while I was among them and, surprisingly, some came to my Bible group. Despite the horrific severity of some of their crimes, it wasn't my place to judge them.

I went about my day as usual, if you could call that usual. We'd just finished morning chow. They'd had to pull Len away from his plate. He was incessantly bashing his head against it. I remembered when they'd first brought him in off the street. He wasn't quite as bad, but now he was over-medicated and worse!

I went back to my cell. I was just starting my prayer/meditation work when Walter came in and said there was supposed to be a laundry exchange soon. As he jumped up on his bunk to take a nap he said he'd just made it back from court and that things hadn't gone well. He was probably burned out from leaving so early in the morning.

I'd meditated for about two hours, and just as I was about to finish, I heard my name over the loudspeakers telling me to, "Roll it up for release!" At least that's what I thought I'd heard. This usually meant you had ten minutes to get all of your property together for release from jail. I was elated! *'Finally, I'm leaving this hellhole! I was innocent in the first place. I should have been gone,'* I thought. Walter woke up at that moment, jumped down from his bunk, and asked if he could have my commissary, sheets, and whatever else I was willing to give away. I was so excited, I started handing things out to whomever came into the cell and asked me.

My name was called again to roll it up. *'Finally!'* I thought. *'They're letting me out of this place.'* When the door opened, the guard motioned for me to come out of the pod to be released. I thanked God at that moment for bringing me safely out of this dreadful place. I was thinking, *'When I'm released, I have nowhere to go. I am officially homeless,'* but I didn't care. I just wanted to be on the street to continue to help others. I thought about the first day I'd arrived there and what it was like to be in hell. But now everything was great because I was officially leaving and all that no longer mattered, despite how bad it was in there.

When I walked out the door, the guard checked my wristband for the last time. "Palmer! Follow me." I didn't look back; I just wanted out of that place. He walked me to another floor, put me in the Recreation room, and told me to wait. An hour passed. Two hours passed. My back was now killing me as I sat on the worn mat on the cold floor. *'That's strange,'* I thought. *'Shouldn't someone have come to pick me up for release at this point? How would I know the standard protocol for release when I've never been in jail before? Let me just relax and wait, no matter how long it takes. At least I'm eventually leaving.'* I kept saying this to myself as the hours drifted by.

Finally, a sheriff came over to bring me chow. I asked him when I was leaving. He pretended not to hear me and walked away. *'That was strange,'* I thought. It was then that they escorted a young black inmate into the room with me. He was very fair-skinned and appeared to be around nineteen. He was dressed in Blues and his hair was all matted together. We spoke a few words, then he went across the room to make a phone call. After talking a few minutes, he suddenly blurted out obscenities to who seemed to be his attorney.

"Damn it! They tricked me!" he yelled.

At this point, he was crying profusely. I went over to him as he hung up the phone and asked if I could help him.

"Nobody can help us. We're going to The Blues!"

I was thinking, 'What does he mean by that?' I knew I was getting ready to go home. I had no idea what had made him say that. I had never seen him before.

Suddenly, he went running across the room over to the mirror above the sink and started bashing his head into it as hard as he could. He wouldn't stop. He screamed at the top of his lungs as he continued to do it. Quickly, I got up, ran over to him, and tried to get him to stop, but he wouldn't. He just kept screaming out, "They're sending us to The Blues!"

I thought, 'The Blues? What is this poor kid talking about?' I thought he was deranged! He continued to yell. Soon the sheriffs came in to restrain him, taking him out and placing him in another room.

Around four hours had now passed. I sat there on a freezing-cold floor and meditated, telling God that whatever was now happening, it was in His hands. Whether I was leaving or not, it was still in His hands. A guard walked over to our doors, opened them, and told us to come with him. The kid started crying again as we lined up single file. The guard came over to me and handed me a pair of Blues.

"No, those aren't for me, sir. There's gotta be some kind of mistake. I'm supposed to be released," I told him.

He ignored me, telling me to hurry up and put them on, then marched us to the elevator.

The kid started screaming, "I told you we were going to The Blues!"

"Faces to the wall!" the guard instructed us.

Those few flights down felt like an airplane in freefall. That's how worn out I was by this time.

"Where are we going, sir?" I asked him politely.

He gave no response. He just repeated for me not to turn around or else he would smash my face! We got off the elevator and he walked us underground through a long tunnel and shouted out to stay on the red line. Finally, we met up with lines of hundreds of other inmates in Blues. We were all merging into one long line. There were about ten guards, all armed with weapons, some semi-automatic. They marched us around bends and down long tunnels until we finally came to an area where they finally separated the kid and me, and gave us a cell number. I was in total shock by this time. I still thought I was leaving. He then started calling out floors.

"Palmer! 2200 floor! Over here in this line!"

Like the kid had said, I wasn't going anywhere soon. I was officially going to the infamous main line. It was time to get prayed up.

BARS FOR STREET WARRIORS

When the guard opened the door, reluctantly I walked in, feeling like I was in Alcatraz. It was old and rundown, and looked like a condemned building with the old-style crank wheel and cable to open the cell door bars. There were two open floors with rows and rows of dingy-green cells as far as one's eyes could see. You could tell they were once a bright orange by the peeling paint on the cell bars. The smell was putrid. It was nauseating.

"Inmate! Your name and cell number!" shouted out the guard on duty.

He repeated it two more times before I responded. I could tell I was making him more agitated by the minute. I had no clue what he wanted me to do. I just stood there and stared into the low-lit cage he was in. It felt like something straight out of a forties prison movie and he was one of the cast of characters. He was clearly an extra, because of where he was pointing for me to walk into; I was sure at any minute I was about to meet the stars of the movie.

He began cranking the old wheel. It screeched as it slowly pulled open the main bars, exposing the row of cells. I walked past his cage reservedly, squinting in the dim lighting to get a glimpse of him. I froze in my steps when I heard the frightening sound of gangs of all races yelling out slogans in different languages and dialects throughout the tier. There was a sea of tattooed hands of all colors without faces extended through cell bars flashing gang signs. There were plastic bags for trash hanging from them. The hypnotic sound of inmates playing tribal beats on the walls was mystifying. It resonated throughout the tiers.

I stepped into the first level and looked above each one for cell 6. I was just trying to buy more time by pretending I was still lost. There was no turning back now, and no way was I going into that cell without first seeing a face, I thought.

"Inmate!" he commanded in a scolding tone. "Lock it down, now!"

His patience had now run thin with me. I still couldn't see who was in the cell; the room was low-lit and felt ominous. It was then that two faces with shifty eyes, both full of harmful intent, appeared out of the cell. One of them motioned for me to step in. I hesitated for a few last precious seconds, like a diver holding his breath just before descending into hell. Cautiously, I stepped in past the cell door. I could hear it being cranked closed behind me. The screeching sound of the wheel was deafening. It was as if it was saying, "Welcome to the hell of all hells!"

I shuddered. I was now trapped and locked in. A sense of claustrophobia came over me as I put my hands to my ears to muffle the sound of it. I looked around the small cell. Vermin were scurrying around under the bunks and everywhere amidst the squalid conditions. The cell contained four rusted bunks and a stainless-steel toilet and sink. There was mold, mildew, and ground-in dirt everywhere, like a sunken ship that had just been raised from the depths of the ocean floor. I had heard that the ACLU had condemned the building years ago. They were now both pointing toward the bunk for me to come sit down between them. It looked like I had no choice at this point, so, in consternation, I obliged them.

Suddenly, I jumped up from the bunk, thinking they were getting ready to rape me (I'd been told the Men's County Jail had one of the highest incidences of rape in the country.) I sized both of them up, and it was obvious they were big enough to overpower me if that was their intention. I was now sweating profusely as I stood there wondering whose idea it had been to put me in this cell with gang members. Dread had now encased me.

"Why're you jumpy, OG?" asked the one inmate.

I didn't answer. I just stood there in mortal shock. Maybe it was my panic anxiety. Maybe it was real. After all, we were in one of the most-notorious jails in the country, where anything could happen at any minute. I just had to be ready to defend myself if it came down to it. I was just the fresh fish in a sea of sharks.

"Sit back down, OG!" the black inmate demanded as he pointed to the area between them on the bunk. I had no choice. Where was I going?

One inmate was a black gang member. He was tall with piercing eyes and neatly-cropped facial hair. The other was a white skinhead. He was short and stubby with gang tattoos all over his head and body. They began asking me all sorts of questions, like where was I from? What was I in for? What was my gang affiliation?

This went on for about an hour. It was intense. I had no idea why all the questions. Finally, they finished and both extended their hands. I exhaled and dropped my head in relief, wondering if I had just passed their rigorous initiation by interrogation.

The skinhead said his name was Jerry the Cutter. I wasn't sure if I should ask him where he'd gotten his name, but I could only guess. The black gang member, who introduced himself as Golo, said he was an L.A. Crip gang member. Even though they both had shaken my hand, I still didn't know whether I should trust them to go to sleep or not. In a shark tank, I knew sleeping fish got eaten, and I knew this jail was full of predators just waiting for you to slip. This place couldn't have earned its infamous reputation based on friendship and kindness.

It was my first night on the main line. I had to stay alert. I had to keep on my guard before I trusted anyone of them. Golo went over to his bunk and began to rap in-sync to a hip-hop beat being played in another cell. The ear-splitting level of the hypnotic groove rang out over the cell tiers as others joined in. He leaned over from his bunk as if checking to see if I liked it. For some reason, I knew the politically correct thing to do was to nod yes. I wasn't ready to piss him off and possibly get in a fight over a rap. The Cutter lay on his bunk, rolled himself a cigarette, and grabbed a book from under his mattress. It was a Bible.

As the night went on, I reached to pull the thin, dingy, worn-out blanket up over me to take the chill off from the frigid cell. There were vermin running around all inside it. Some of them were jumping out of the air vent of the musty cell to grab the leftovers from night chow. The smell was putrid and nauseating. Golo and The Cutter seemed oblivious to it; they never flinched or commented about it as they prepared for bed. They were clearly institutionalized. As I lay there I could hear inmates arguing about the Top Ramen noodles owed to them by other inmates and how they would get a beat down if they didn't pay them. Their tense voices echoed across rows of cells as the tensions quickly mounted. You could feel it as it rolled in across the tiers like an enigmatic fog over the San Francisco Bay at dusk.

Just as I was almost asleep, I was jolted awake by the sudden loud words of, "Radio! Radio!" filling the space (a radio was a message for every race in the dorm to be silent and respect the leader from the gang who was talking). It was spoken by a Crip gang leader. With the tiers now silent, the leader began to shout out gang slogans that came off just as in-sync as a Marine marching band. The entire tier soon joined in with him, including Golo, who was rattling the bars and reciting the slogans in full voice with their leader. He then instructed the black gang members—everyone in his gang—to shut it down for the evening. Within seconds, the entire tier of Crips were quieter than monks in a monastery.

Throughout this entire time, you weren't allowed to flush toilets or talk; those were grounds for getting seriously DP'd (disciplined). Next, the Woods (the whites and skinheads) leader yelled out a few gang slogans and was soon followed by a revelry of white inmates, the same way as with the Crips. I could hear the Woods in all the cells and tiers above us joining in. The Cutter (the white skinhead) in our cell now joined in. Finally, the Southsiders (the Mexicans) gang leader shouted out slogans in Spanish that were much longer and more intense than the others.

Soon the room was in total silence. Once the gang rituals were done, there were no voices heard in the cells, only whispers, until the next morning. It was the strict rule. That would be grounds for a serious beat down (DP). Golo said this was done 365 days a year. The gang politics in the Blues between the races were very serious. I was told that everyone in the Yellows avoided being sent to the main line, the Blues, at all cost. It was said that some men faked being psychotic, faked depression, and cried like babies when they heard they were being sent here. This was the hellhole of all hells, it was said.

Things finally died down after the radio. I tried to sleep, but the sound of hip-hop beats banging relentlessly on the hollows of the walls prevented it. I was restless the entire time as I lay there and thought about my family. I began to think about all the families of the other inmates. What could I do to help? There's gotta be something I can do to make a difference. *'God, you gave me a gift. I just have to be brave enough here in order to use it. I have to trust in You.'* I was now in a darker world, and I knew the kind of strength to survive spiritually in here would take a lot. I was now amongst the toughest, most intimidating in society. I just had to remember those three words I'd vowed earlier—no more fear!

DEFINE BRAVE

The next morning, I went to court. The judge asked if I still wanted to continue to take it all the way to trial. I told him yes. This meant the next appearance would be the pretrial. The woman whose home I'd gone into would be there for the first time to give her version of the story on that night. I just hoped it would be the truth. I knew she was probably still devastated, and there wasn't a night I didn't pray for her and her son.

My attorney advised me not to chance it. The entire time he'd had represented me, he hadn't known anything about my career in the music industry. I'd only told him I was homeless. My family had begged me to tell him; they felt it might help my case. I told them I understood, but I was doing God's work in there and who I'd been prior to this didn't matter. It had been months now and my joint pain had not returned—not even once! It was truly a miracle, and I shared with them that that was the promise I'd made to God in exchange for it. They were stunned because they all knew what I'd endured for years. I told them I was on a low dosage med for the depression and it was working, but what really helped, I believed, was that I was too busy doing God's work to even notice it. It was cathartic.

Being incarcerated had shown me firsthand how inmates of low socioeconomic status, especially those of color, were given unreasonably long sentences. I was now preaching to these same inmates. Why should I be a hypocrite and use my resumé to get a better deal than them? The godly spirit growing in me wouldn't let me do it, I told them. It made them very sad, but said they respected what I was standing for. I understood they were scared for my safety, but I assured them that their faith in God was watching over me.

When I returned from court that day, I was moved from the cell with Golo and Jerry, and we said our goodbyes. By this time, I had been moved around the jail system several times. I never knew what I was going to face whenever I arrived at a new pod, only that it could be just as dangerous as the last. The moment you entered a new environment, you were starting over. That could be good or terrible, but I knew the comforting spirit of God was with me always, and in knowing that, I had no fear.

This particular one had two levels, and the day room and tables were in the center. Because of the overcrowding, inmate bunks filled the entire area. It took a few days for me to settle in and get a feel for the pod. There was always an inmate who ran it, and you had to make sure you didn't get in his way or even make him feel in the slightest way that that was your intention. That's just how it was in jail. Each dorm leader had his own set of rules and plenty of enforcers around to do his bidding if you disrupted it.

After a few days had passed, I decided to try to start a new prayer group. Some of the inmates were going around begging for coffee shots, others were gambling in the corner, and others watching TV. I looked around for willing inmates to join the table. A few Latino Southsiders and other inmates came when suddenly, from the top level behind me, I heard this loud voice yell out, "If anyone wants to challenge me, I'll meet you under the staircase!"

It was Leo. He chose that area because all the inmates knew where the camera's blind spots were, so if there was going to be a stabbing or a fight, it wouldn't be caught on camera. No one took Leo up on his offer. It was easy to see why: he was at least six-foot-seven and would tip the scale at well over three hundred pounds. He yelled out again, but this time he added, "Whoever meets me there won't be coming out." He made it clear that he was a lifer, with nothing to lose if he killed you. This went on every day for weeks.

When the nurses would come to the pods to give out meds through the flap in the door, we'd have to line up on the staircase. Well, Leo didn't like that because he felt that he didn't need to get in the line. He would always stand at the top of the landing, and if an inmate got in front of him at the bottom of the staircase, it could easily turn fatal for them. Most inmates abided by that rule. Leo ran that pod.

One day, I went to the door to see how far down the row of other pods the nurse was. Leo somehow mistook that as me jumping in front of him in the line. He went ballistic. He started screaming at me, "How dare you cut in front of me! I run this pod!"

I had no clue what he was talking about. The entire pod went silent at that moment. I'm not sure I wanted to even turn around, but I did. Was I afraid? At first—yes. But I knew I was there to do God's work, so I walked up the stairs and stood in front of him. I looked straight up his body which towered over me, and into his eyes. I'm sure every inmate in that room thought that he was going to throw me over the railing at any moment.

But I saw something different. I saw a man whose spirit was lost and needed God to help him find it. He then repeated what he'd said, only hollering even louder, despite me now extending my hand for him to shake. He refused.

"Where'd you get the guts to come up to me like this?" he asked. "What if I threw your ass over this rail?"

He then had a puzzled look on his face. God was telling me that he was a broken soul, and this was why He wanted me to talk to him. So, I told him it wasn't bravery, it was faith.

"True power isn't in how you threaten people here. True power is in taking up for the ones being threatened," I shared with him.

A sad look spread across Leo's face and he apologized. He then explained to me why he was such an angry person.

"Preach, one day I went to my best friend's house. He had betrayed me on a drug deal that had gone bad and he kept my money. When he answered the door, he knew why I was there and was expecting me. He pulled a gun out from behind his back and told me to get on my knees, and when I did, he put it in my mouth and pulled the trigger. That was all I remembered. A month later, I woke up in the hospital, and noticed I had a hole in the roof of my mouth the size of a nickel, and two shattered bullets protruding out the back of my skull where they had lodged."

He opened his mouth and pointed to it, then turned around to show me the back of his head, where the skin had grown over them. He said that when he finally got out of the hospital he went back to his friend's house, and when he opened the door he blew the man's brains out.

"So, Preach, when you see me get a little crazy, I really don't mean to. They got me on these strong meds, and sometimes they just don't work."

I told him I understood. The rest of my time in that pod, Leo would always come down from his perch at the end of my prayer group and lean over the table. He'd then put his long-reaching arms around all of us as we prayed. I was very moved, how a man who had killed now wanted to know more about God, redemption, and grace. He no longer wanted to be a bully, or a victim, because of his mental state. Once again, I was learning how fragile we all are, and it doesn't take much to break that thread.

CALL YOUR SISTER

"Laundry! Line it up for laundry exchange!" came the call over the intercom. That usually happened once a week, depending on what pod you were in or what mood the guards were in. We lined up at the door, then walked out and entered the halls where the guards and trustees stood to exchange items with us for clean blue jail garments, a white tee-shirt, and bright neon-green boxers.

As I got closer in the line, an inmate behind me asked my name. I told him it was Robert Palmer, but the inmates called me Preach.

"Nice to meet you. My name is Stephen, but everyone calls me Steve."

Steve was white and about five-four. You could tell he must have recently been arrested because his hair looked freshly cut and his fingers were still manicured.

"Do you have an extra blanket I can buy?"

I told him I'd give him one for free, but he didn't believe me. He knew there had to be a catch, because everything in jail costs. When we returned to the jail dorm, he came over and I gave him one. It's impolite to ask an inmate what he's in for. Sometimes, one will voluntarily tell you. Also, until they've gone to trial and are sentenced, everything is an allegation. Steve went on about his meth use and how he was trying to quit. He said he came from a very prominent family but he was always in and out of jail. He was an outcast because of it. I told him I did most of the prayer work with the inmates, and if he ever needed any, he was welcome to come to me or the prayer group.

"I used to know that Book inside and out!" he suddenly blurted out in reference to the Bible.

"What happened?" I asked him.

"He kept letting me down. Yeah, that's what it was. That's when I turned to drugs. I love the high meth gives me. It lets me escape from the world. It doesn't ask me questions, just treats me nice."

That's when I told him about my drug use back in the days before my heart attack. How I'd taken God out of my life, and later, overdosed and died. It was He who'd brought me back. How I'd become depressed and recently tried to take my life. Once again, He was there and had delivered me from it. That was how I was able to preach the Word in jail about the salvation and redemption He offers us all.

"I don't know, Preach. I don't mean no disrespect, but you gotta know I've heard all that before. I'm pretty much over that kind of preaching. It doesn't do anything for me."

I told him that would never stop God from loving him. He just laughed and went and stood over in line for chow. Later that night during Bible study, I noticed Steve kept walking by and stopping for a few minutes, then he'd hurry and walk away. I was hoping he was still curious.

When I finished for the night, he came over and asked if I would let him have a Snickers bar until he got his commissary. I had him follow me over to my cell.

"Preach, I overheard you preaching to the inmates. I remember every word you read from the Bible. I just wish it still had the same meaning for me, but it doesn't. Now it just seems like a lot of words."

"Steve, I understand how you could feel like that, but the meaning will never change. I found, in times of my life when I thought I didn't need God, there was usually something I was doing that was keeping me from the edification of His Word. In my case, as in yours, it was drugs. It was diluting His message to a point where it didn't have any meaning at all. And without any meaning, it couldn't help me get through the tough times. After a while I just totally gave up on God. I blamed Him."

The lights were now starting to dim in the jail pod, bringing our night to an end.

"Preach, I'll think about what you said when I get back over to my bunk. Thanks for the words. Being in here this time just might be a good thing for me. Maybe it was God this time that put you in here to tell me those words, especially like you said, when the mind is clouded by things like meth we can't understand His Word or see how much He loves us."

I knew it was God who'd put me there for him. There was something life-altering awaiting him that he needed to prepare for.

"Chow! Wake up for chow!" came the early-morning sound blaring over the loudspeakers the next day. I got in the long line behind Steve.

"Hey! Good morning, Preach. How'd you sleep?"

"It was pretty good. I meditated for a few hours before finally drifting off."

"What time is your Bible study today?"

"About four. It depends on what the inmates are doing at that time."

"Oh, okay."

"Do I sense you getting interested?" I jokingly said to him.

"I'm just curious, that's all. We'll see."

I was glad Steve was maybe starting to come around. We finished eating and I went back to my cell to prepare for the first one.

There were several phones in the pod located right next to the Spyder tables. During my Bible study, Steve walked over to the one next to our table. I didn't notice him at first, until he got really loud and started cursing at someone on the line.

"I don't have to take this s*** from you or anyone else in this family!" he blurted out.

An inmate at our table threatened to beat him up if he didn't respect what we were doing there. I told him it was all right; he probably just was going through something. Steve overheard the inmate, then lowered his voice, but whoever he was talking to, you could tell it was still heated. It went on for a while longer, and by the time he hung up, my Bible study had ended. He walked up to my cell and asked if it was okay to come in. I nodded.

"Hey, Preach, I'm sorry for what happened earlier; that was really embarrassing."

"No reason to apologize, Steve; things happen. If there's anything you ever want to talk about, always know I'm here for you with prayer."

"Thanks, Preach; that means a lot. My sister and I have been fighting for years, especially since I started doing drugs pretty heavy. She told me our mom just got admitted to the hospital. They're not sure yet what's wrong with her. They're gonna keep her for a few days for observation."

"Wow! I hope she's all right. We'll keep her in prayer tonight."

"Thanks, I'd really appreciate that. That's very kind of you guys."

After that, Steve returned to the dorm to call his sister back.

When I came back out for Bible study with the inmates, he was on the phone arguing with her again. This time he lowered his voice when he saw we were about to start, but it didn't stop him from quarreling with her. When he finally got off the phone I motioned for him to come over and pray with us as we approached the end. Reluctantly, he did. Afterward, he followed me and talked to me while I put the Bibles back under my bunk.

"Do you still have one?" I asked him.

"No, I misplaced it years ago, but I betcha I can still quote any Scripture you pull up. That I can still do," he said, a sense of pride in his voice.

"Okay, tell me about the parable of the lost sheep.'"

He quoted it almost word-for-word.

"Steve, that's very impressive, but I think what's more important is, do you remember what it means?"

"How the Pharisees couldn't understand how Christ ate with sinners and He told them, 'Rejoice with Me. I have found my lost sheep. I tell you that in the same way there will be more rejoicing in heaven over one sinner who repents than over ninety-nine righteous persons who do not need to repent.'"

I can tell he was touched by it and maybe it left a small opening for God to come back in. It was great to see it all coming back to him. I said a prayer for Steve that night. God told me not to give up on him. I knew entirely too well what he was going through. I'd been there myself, trying to find a place in the glass of life to put God, when it was already full to the brim with things that were destroying it. Do we have to experience a disaster first for God to get our attention? Steve's awakening was just around the corner.

When I walked out into the pod that afternoon, Steve was back on the phone, arguing with his sister. When he got off this time, I told him I had something important to tell him.

"Steve, when I prayed for you last night—I know you might not believe what I'm about to tell you, but God showed me a vision for you."

"Really? What's that?"

"He told me to tell you to make up with your sister and talk to your mom. It's very important for you too."

"Preach, I'm very confused. *Why?*"

"I'm not sure yet, but you should call her back now and make up with her."

I knew he was confused and it probably didn't make any sense what I'd just told him, because it didn't make any sense to me yet. He went over and called her, and I could see for the first time that he wasn't screaming at her. She let him talk to his mom. When he came back over, I noticed he was clutching his Bible. He asked if I would pray with him. He felt lost. I did as he requested, but I knew God was telling him something he needed to hear.

"Preach, it was nice to finally make peace with my sister and finally get to talk to my mom after all this time. It's been a while. She sounded great!"

Later that day, I called Steve over. I told him I believed the reason God wanted him to make peace with his sister and talk to his mom was because she was going to die that week.

"No way!" he shouted.

I took him into my cell to avoid riling up the dorm. "Steve, when God gives me these kinds of visions, I just try to prepare whoever it is for. It's rare I get this kind. Very rare. But I'm sure it's accurate. For your sake, I hope it's not."

He sat there on my bunk and cried. I tried to console him. I prayed with him into the night to try to help him understand that we never know when God wants to bring one of us home, how this place was a temporary home for us all, and that if he and his mom believed in God they would share everlasting life with Him. That's why it is so important to accept Him. He asked if he could sleep in the vacant bunk below me. I told him it was fine. He woke me up several times in the night to pray for his mother.

That next morning, he was on the phone and I could tell it was his sister by the conversation. Then out of nowhere, he yelled out, "No! Not Mom! She can't be dead!" He dropped the phone and just stared at me. I couldn't even imagine what he was going through at that moment. He was in such shock he just walked away from the phone, forgetting his sister was still on it, and just broke down in the dorm. Quickly, I took him to my cell and sat him on the bed.

"Preach, there's just no way you could've known that," he said.

The tears were pouring down his face. I gave him some toilet paper and asked him to pull out his Bible. I read him a few Scriptures and held him while I prayed for him. His spirit was broken. Still crying, he lifted his head up and told me, "These past few years, especially after I got addicted to drugs, my mom and I weren't very close, but I guess it's a blessing I got to speak to her before she died. That is simply amazing. I just can't believe you saw that. It's hard to believe she's gone."

Steve went in and called his sister back. When he came back, she'd told him she was sad their mom had suddenly died, but she was so happy he'd gotten a chance to make peace with her beforehand. Their mom had gotten to see them make up, which also made her very happy.

Steve came to my cell every day after that for Bible study. He put in for an early release to go to his mother's funeral. I'm not sure if they granted it to him because a few days later my name was called to transfer to another dorm. When Steve heard the news, he ran over to me. I knew he was still very fragile.

"Steve, I feel God's is telling me my job here is done. I believe it was only to bring you back to Him, the lost sheep, remember? To prepare you for life's unexpected. Keep Him close to you, my friend, and He'll always be your comforting guide. I've learned that from experience."

We hugged and he walked me to the door. Little did I know God had tragic news waiting for me just around the corner.

It's About The Truth

I'd spoken to my family late that night and told them I'd call when I got back from court. Today was another court day. I was looking forward to this one because I knew that the judge's decision was crucial. The past few visits, he'd said I could walk if I was willing to take a felony strike. But I intended to pass as usual simply because I was innocent.

When we arrived at court that morning, I felt anxious knowing this judge could be as harsh as usual. I didn't expect him to offer me a better deal, not that day or any other for that matter. The bus pulled into the court parking area at about 7:30 a.m. We unloaded, walked down the gradient, and were checked in by the waiting sheriffs before being escorted to our waiting tanks.

I sat there contemplating my fate—not just here, but my life in general. What would I do when I eventually left that horrid place? Probably get back to my relationship with my family, especially my mom. I'd had a dream about her that told me she was going to die very soon. This saddened my spirit, knowing how close I was to her. I quickly had to bring myself back to my immediate reality and focus on my trial. Hours later, a sheriff came and escorted some of us to the cells up on the court floors. That was usually where you waited to meet your attorney before going in front of the judge.

A few more hours passed and I was brought into the cubicle, facing my attorney behind the glass. He seemed spry and in a good mood. He gave me an update concerning my trial. Nothing had changed other than a new judge was taking over my case. That could be good or prove disastrous; only time would tell. I told him, when he went in, to tell the judge, "Don't get me wrong, my freedom means a lot to me, but my dignity and honor mean more. That's why I won't take the deal he's offering."

We were now in-sync and ready to face the judge. Today was my pretrial. The woman whose house I'd gone into would take the stand today. I felt so sorry for her and her son. I couldn't imagine how traumatic that incident had been for them. Maybe that was why she'd trumped up the incident of what really happened. I was sure the police had told her to add more to get a stronger conviction. It was the moment I'd been waiting for. Hopefully, since time had passed, it had given her time to consider telling the truth about what really had happened that night, not the story she'd given the sheriffs when she'd gone on record.

She had alleged that I had gone into her home and menaced her family with a knife. Anyone who knew me knew that just wasn't possible. I simply was not that kind of person, and there were plenty of people who lived in the building who'd said they were willing to testify to it. I was praying she would tell the truth so I could be released with just a misdemeanor. I knew I wouldn't get the chance to tell her I was sorry because she'd had a restraining order put out on me a few months back.

After a few minutes, I was cuffed and led into the courtroom. This was my first time seeing the poor woman since the night of the incident. I couldn't apologize enough in my spirit for it. I was now reliving the moment that night I'd tried to commit suicide. It was haunting me as I sat there and watched her approach the stand. The story she gave of the night of the incident once again, unfortunately, wasn't true. I was very disappointed in her testimony. I knew I had been wrong for entering her home, but she should have told the real story of what had happened. I imagined she had been coached with her statement.

I jumped up in the middle of the courtroom and told my attorney she wasn't telling the truth. He told me to stay calm and wait for my chance in the actual trial. I felt let down by the system. It was that easy to make up a story and put a man behind bars. I was stunned. So, I was guilty until proven innocent? That just didn't make much sense to me.

The judge told me he was astonished I wasn't in a hurry to leave the hardcore inmates I was in jail with. Little did he know, I followed wherever God led me now. My case was no longer important; I felt they'd already made their minds up anyway. He just stared at me, shaking his head in disbelief. He went off the record and told me he'd never had a case such as mine.

After we left the courtroom, my attorney again tried convincing me to take the deal that was offered. Once again, I told him no way. I told him I wanted to go to trial, whether I won or lost. If I lost I would face a possible four-year sentence in a penitentiary. I didn't care about the consequences. My faith was strong. I knew the Holy Spirit would guide me to the right decision. I was very frustrated and wanted to go back to county jail to finish my spiritual work.

The judge had made it clear I could walk if I was willing to take his deal. I made the tough decision to stay in county jail and ignore my trial. I prayed on it and now it was in the Holy Spirit's hands. I had officially and spiritually released myself from the burden of it. The only thing on my mind was servitude to the inmates. In my heart I felt that I could make a difference. I was now more committed than ever.

I boarded the sheriff's bus and headed back to jail. On the way back, all I could think of was the spiritual work I was doing back at County. I could now focus solely on the inmates. Was I ready to take possibly four years for not settling for the deal that was offered? My faith was about to be tested. If I lost in court, was I willing to continue doing my work with the inmates regardless of where they sent me?

I opened my Bible to the book of Acts to read how Paul had learned to trust God, no matter the consequences. I needed that kind of strength. When faced with adversity, you have to turn it over to God and stick hard to what you believe, even if it means your life. There was a lesson I felt God was trying to teach me. My faith in Him is what kept me going. I now knew what I'd taken on was far greater and more significant than my own freedom.

GOD SAID TO KEEP HER

I was halfway into my morning meditation, which was very important for me. It brought me so much closer to God—the peace and tranquility—and it also kept my mind off the depression. The suicidal thoughts were gone, and lately I felt I had reached a milestone with it. Other than that, which was a lot, it was just another usual day in the jail dorm. We were always on lockdown, twenty-four/seven, with no windows. There were a lot of felons and three-strikers facing long sentences for murder. Then there were the inmates getting disciplined in a corner by at least twenty of their own gang members, simply because they hadn't done their morning push-ups or taken a shower. Or, a shakedown of the dorm because of a suspected shank. The list went on and on.

I'd noticed for the past few days, around the same time, an inmate who would walk by, stop right in the middle of my cell and start rapping loudly. I could tell he was into Lil Wayne, the rapper. I happened to like some of his material as well, just not so much the ones filled with too many expletives. I'd overheard other inmates call him Junie. This went on for about a week, and by this point, during my meditations, I started to wonder what God was telling me. Was there a reason why He was sending him in front of me, unknown to even Junie himself... yet?

A few days later, while I meditated, he walked by rapping as usual. But this morning was different. Right when he got in front of me, he suddenly stopped rapping and tapped my bunk. I opened my eyes and he introduced himself. Standing in front of me was this six-foot-eight, handsome young man, with a hearty grin.

"Hi. I know they call you Preach, right? I see you sitting here every day, meditating for hours, then you go and pray, then study with the other inmates. Tell me how you can sit here almost the entire day and meditate with all this noise going on?"

I told him it took a lot of discipline, and if he wanted to learn, I'd teach him.

"Preach, I don't know if I'm quite ready for all that yet, but I did tell my girlfriend about you 'cause she's really into God. We recently started dating, just before I was picked up and arrested on another drug charge and being in a gang, which I know she hates. The judge said I might be facing a lot of years this time. She said she'd still wait for me. Anyway, the reason I'm here talking to you is because she was trying to get me into God before I got arrested. I'm not sure if this whole God thing is for me yet, but I'm willing to try, for her."

"What's her name?"

"Her name's Regina, Regina Morrison."

"That's a beautiful name, Junie. I know you might not believe what I'm about to tell you, but hopefully, in time, you will. God reveals everything in His time, and I'm sure He's trying to tell you and Regina something? These next few days, why don't you come by in the mornings and let me pray with you and help you learn more about how much we all really need Him in our lives?"

Reluctantly, Junie agreed to try it and came by most of that next week. Before heading back to his bunk one morning, he looked as if something was bothering him.

"Junie, are you okay?" I asked.

"No, Preach. Regina's starting to get on my nerves again. She's pushing this God thing too hard on me. I think I'm gonna break up with her, maybe tonight. I really don't want to, because I truly love her, but it's getting to be way too much for me."

"Junie, maybe now wouldn't be the right time to do that. Give it some more time."

He told me he didn't feel he had a choice at this point, because God wasn't important enough to make him stay, and that was her thing, not his. He headed over to the phones, and just before he dialed, I yelled out one last time for him not to do it. I just knew I needed to fight for her. He was now talking to her and suddenly gave a thumbs up to indicate that he hadn't done it.

'Whew!' I thought. 'God really had His hands on this.' I waved as a sign of relief.

The night was now coming to an end. I did my meditation and prayer before turning in. Most of the dorm had already gone to sleep as I lay there waiting myself. There was a cold chill in the room and most inmates had thin blankets pulled up over them. God came to me and said, "Walk to the end of the dorm, then turn around, and at that moment, Junie, who is now asleep, will sit up in his bunk, confused, not knowing why he woke up. Then tell him what I'm instructing you to do now, and the reason he sat up in his bunk is a sign from Me for him to keep Regina close. Robert, for those who don't know Me, I still know and love them, and want so much for this one to know Me as well."

I did as He told me. I got up and walked past Junie, who was in a deep sleep, and went to the end of the dorm. I turned and, miraculously, he sat up, looking confused as he scratched his head. I went up to him and asked if he knew why he'd just woken up.

"No," he said. "That's really strange. I was in a deep sleep, and suddenly, I saw a light. Then I woke up, and now I'm just sitting here scratching my head. Wow, that's crazy."

When I told him what God had instructed me to do, I'm not sure whether he believed it or not, but he knew something was unusual about it. I then prayed with him to release inside himself whatever was holding him back from accepting God's love and not run from it, as I'd once done when I tried to kill myself. I had no idea what he'd gone through in his life, but it must've been hard. I begged him once again to stay with Regina. We both then turned in for the night.

That next morning was a typical day, until the jail dorm gang leader yelled out my name from across the dorm.

"Preach! I need you now!"

I jumped up and ran over to him. When I got there, he looked at me with sadness on his face and said,

"Preach, this is over my head." Junie was sitting there, crying inconsolably, with a friend trying to comfort him. He wouldn't let anyone help him.

"What happened?" I asked his friend.

"Preach, Junie's got three kids and two of them live in South Carolina. His son, William, is seven, and his daughter, Sheana, is eight. They were at home with his ex-girlfriend's boyfriend, who was babysitting them for her. Junie's son was playing karate in the room, when the boyfriend asked him to stop. The son told him he didn't have to because it wasn't his house. The boyfriend got mad and smacked him, hard." His son fell backwards down a flight of stairs, broke his neck, and now lay there, dead. His neck was broken. The boyfriend then panicked and ran from the house, leaving the sister there alone. He was nowhere to be found.

"Preach, please help him?" his friend, cried out hopelessly.

I now saw that God's plan was to bring Regina into Junie's life and make sure I fought hard to keep her there. I took his hand and helped him up. He was a mess. I couldn't possibly understand what was going through his mind. His heart must have felt like it had been torn from his body. I walked him back to his bunk, and as we walked through the dorm of one hundred and fifty inmates, they were all speechless as they mourned for him. The silence in the room was deafening. No loud card games were going in the background from an inmate cheating. No sports were blaring from the TV. No gang-bangers were stomping each other out in the corner. They were all in observance of Junie's loss. It could have been one of their own kids.

It was all on God right now. He was the center of attention. We sat there on Junie's bunk. I put his head in my lap and held him tightly, as if he were my own son. I just let him cry it out while I prayed for him in only a whisper that he could hear: "Dear Father God, this lost young man lying here wants to know You, but doesn't quite know how. His spirit has been broken, and only You can assuage and heal it. I am only Your messenger who has made this union possible, and now, please let him see and feel the awesome power of the God I know and have witnessed in my own life."

We sat there for hours and hours as he continued to cry. Then, as if he'd been baptized in holy water straight from the River Jordan, Junie raised his head up, looked at me, and said, "Preach, I'm good. I don't quite know why. I'm still really hurting. It's a pain I've never felt before and I miss my son, William so much already, but I'm good. I don't know how long it's going to last, but He touched something inside me that gave me peace."

I was witnessing nothing less than a miracle. Only hours previously, Junie's son was lying at the foot of those stairs, his poor little neck broken and his life taken from him. Junie was never going to see him again. Yet he reassured me again, then got up, went over to the basketball area and joined in a game. All of his friends came over to cheer him on for his amazing strength.

Later that night, he came over to tell me he'd spoken to Regina, who I couldn't help but remember. It had been less than a week since he'd wanted to break up with her because she was trying to push God onto him. Now that same amazing, God-sent woman was about to catch a late flight, all because his son's mother couldn't be found. She was going there to do everything she could to bring his daughter to stay with her. She was certain God had put her in his life just for this. She also told him that his ex-girlfriend's brother had found the boyfriend later and killed him.

"Preach, she always said to me that God worked in mysterious ways."

That's when I told him that if he was still on the outside when it had happened, he might have gone there and killed him. He said it probably would have happened that way.

"I do believe her now. I've learned a lot from this. For the first time in my life I actually prayed on my own last night. I prayed for Him to show me how to do this. After losing my son I'm through with gangs. I think it was a sign for me to start doing right. Regina said, no matter how many years I get, she will wait for me and marry me when I get out."

I was so happy for them.

Unfortunately, that next week my time came to leave, just when we were making so much progress. That day, as I meditated before leaving, I told God I didn't understand why He was taking me away from him so soon. "What if he isn't ready?" He told me He only needed me to bring him inside the gate and He would always take care of him from here. His words always seemed to give me comfort, especially in moments like this, when I was at a loss to understand.

Walking out the door, I went to look for him to say goodbye. Another inmate said he was in the restroom. I walked over, and just as I was about to walk in, I overheard him telling another inmate how sad he was, because God had put this man in his life and now He was taking him away. He was having a hard time understanding it. For some reason, I couldn't walk in to say goodbye. It would have been too painful for the both of us. Something wouldn't let me do it. So, I went to the front door and waited for the guard to unlock it, to let me out, to go to another dorm in the jail, to start this process all over again—recruiting broken souls and bringing them to the only One I knew who could save them.

My work was done there. Junie, Regina, and his daughter Sheana were going to be all right. God bless them and his lost son William.

A Troubled Spirit

It was on a Thursday, in the early part of the evening. I knew I was destined to meet Truman. I knew there was something different about him from the thirty-odd new fish who had just come into the jail dorm at that moment. He was black, tall, and looked to be about forty. He had a low-key, quiet demeanor about himself, and was exceptionally-dark skinned. It glistened off the lights in the room like a lacquered-black piano.

He stood there with his bedroll under his arm as the head rep for the dorm started handing out bunk assignments. Of all the available ones in the dorm, I knew he would be next to mine. God had plans unknown to him at that moment. Within minutes after going around the large dorm, he was finally directed to bunk number 36. One hundred and fifty bunks in the room filled with inmates, and the one to my right, bunk number 36, was the one he was assigned to. He was being led to where he needed to be.

I closed my eyes to finish my evening prayer/meditation work. After a few minutes, I was disrupted by someone with a strong southern drawl tapping on my bunk to get my attention. I opened my eyes and it was him.

"Hi, my name is Truman, Truman Mitchell," he said as he extended his hand to greet me. "They told me this bunk next to you is number thirty-six."

I nodded my head and asked him if he needed help getting settled in. He reminded me of a southern gentleman out of an old Sidney Poitier movie. He had calloused hands and a very firm handshake.

"Good to meet you, my brother. I'm Robert Palmer, but here they call me Preach. I minister and help a lot of the inmates in here."

Truman climbed up onto his bunk and began making it up meticulously. I wondered if he'd been in the military. After about half-an-hour, the sheriff ordered us via the loudspeakers to get ready for chow.

"Are you hungry?" I asked him.

"I'm starving, Preach," he said as he folded the last part of the sheet perfectly over on his bunk. He asked if I was an ordained minister.

"No, I'm just one of God's faithful servants," I told him as the food cart pulled up to us. I frowned in repugnance at the disgusting dinner tray.

"Here, take my milk," Truman offered as he nodded approvingly to what I'd just told him. He said he thought it was great I'd taken such an interest in the inmates. "Nobody else cares about us," he said as he took another bite of his breaded-chicken patty.

I told him I did, and maybe being in here was my true calling (I didn't tell him or any other inmate about my background in the entertainment industry — if they asked, I simply said I was homeless and had come off the streets, which at that point was true).

Truman asked how long I'd been in the dorm. I told him I'd been there for months fighting my case, and I did prayer work with inmates of all ethnicities and religions. He was shocked. He said he found it strange that I could meditate in the middle of the room from my bunk with all the constant commotion in the dorm. I told him it wasn't easy, and it had taken time learning how to do it.

"I have no judgment when it comes to why the inmates are here," I told him.

"What about the strict politics in here?"

I told him they existed but I followed my spirit. It told me to give words of comfort to anyone who asked, regardless of their alleged crime, and that was why I did it. Truman told me I was bold. We both laughed. Little did he know I would be bringing him something he needed before the evening was out. He continued to laugh as we put our empty food trays on the pile with the others. We then headed back to our bunks. On the way we passed Sean, a white skinhead who was facing several years for alleged meth drug trafficking. I introduced him to Truman.

"How's your trial going?" I asked Sean.

"Preach, I just got sentenced yesterday," he said. "Your praying with me the night before I went in really helped calm my nerves. I took a plea bargain and settled for five years. They're sending me to San Quentin later this month. I can't wait to get there so I can get out of this hellhole. Keep praying for me, Preach," he hollered as we walked away.

"Preach, they seem like they really rely on your words of comfort in here," Truman observed.

I told him I enjoyed doing it. It was one of the most gratifying things I'd ever done in my life. He probably had no idea how chaotic my life in the entertainment industry was before I'd gotten here.

We walked further down and ran into Creeper, a Southsider gang member from East L.A. He was sitting at the edge of his bunk, making a beautiful cross necklace out of Skittles wrappers. What was he doing in this terrible place with so much talent? His case was one I really couldn't understand. He was facing a life sentence for the murder of a rival gang member. It was his third strike. He had come to me a month earlier asking for prayer for him and his family. I had spoken to his wife a few days earlier to renew her confidence in God. She and their family were relieved. I asked him if they'd offered him a deal yet. He said fifty years was the best they'd come back with so far.

"Are you gonna take it?" I asked him.

"I need prayers from you, Preach. Is it cool if I come to your bunk later tonight?"

I told him it was fine as he nodded and hugged me.

We finally arrived back at the bunks. I noticed something wasn't right with Truman as he stood between them, staring at the ceiling and fidgeting. Something was seriously bothering him. I could feel it in my spirit, and it was becoming more evident by the minute. I asked him if he wanted to talk about it, but he said he was fine. It was time for my Bible study with the inmates. They were gathering around our bunk, but God was telling me Truman needed it more than any of them at that moment.

"Hey, Preach, I see these guys in here seem really comfortable talking to you about their lives," Truman remarked.

"I think, over a short period of time I've gained their trust, and for it I am so humbly grateful," I answered, pointing my finger around at the group.

"Preach, he doesn't take us for granted," they told him.

"You can come to him at any time of the day or night, seven days a week, and he's there for you. If you need clothes, blankets, food or prayer, Preach has got your back," Thomas shouted out (if convicted, he was facing a life sentence for a double homicide).

It was then that Truman began to open up about growing up in the south and how tough it had been for him as a kid. He talked about his case and what he was in for. "Petty stuff!" he shouted, but we could see on his face that something deeper was troubling him.

"Hey, Preach, why don't you talk to your new buddy here tonight alone? We can come back later or tomorrow if you want," Jason suggested.

Jason was a Korean gang member facing hard time for repeated burglaries. The others looked at each other and agreed with him. I looked over at Truman, and he nodded back in agreement. All the guys in my different Bible study groups could feel when an inmate needed a one-on-one. They were all used to it by now. They started to disperse, going back to their bunks for the night. Most were waiting for their transfers, but none knew when. They could be called at any second over the loudspeakers to roll it up. Some were worried, knowing that if convicted they soon would be transferred to a prison to serve out long sentences (for some, possibly life). They were all on edge most of the time.

That was why I believed some came to me, feeling maybe God was the answer after all this time. God had put me in the right place to try to help them spiritually before they left. Knowing this, I knew Truman could be leaving at any minute, so I felt a strong urge to talk to him before he left. Every minute wasted was precious.

Soon, over the loudspeakers, came the order to return to our bunks and lock it down for the night. For a few extra minutes we stood there as inmates walked by to say their goodnights, then we sat on our bunks to talk. The noise in the dorm was now beginning to subside and that's when Truman told me there was something he wanted to discuss. He hadn't felt comfortable with the group around, and wanted to talk privately. An hour had passed and it was now the time they usually called out names to roll it up for transfer. You could hear it blaring over the loudspeakers. Whew! Truman wasn't called out in the first batch, but I knew it was now or never; if I didn't speak with him right then he would soon be leaving. Something in my spirit told me he needed it badly.

In those next few hours, Truman finally began to open up. I was absolutely stunned by the things that had happened in his life, but it felt like he'd left out something vital that he really wanted to share. I was certain of it. I closed my eyes and began to talk to him. I told him how his toughness was a smokescreen to protect the little boy inside him. Because of this, he felt he'd become a killing machine for the Army when necessary. Any time his inner child felt threatened, he would react with violence, and deep down inside himself, he didn't understand this. It was God's words coming to me that I shared with him. After I was finished, about an hour later, I had only a partial recollection of what I'd said to him.

When it was done, I opened my eyes and looked at Truman. I could feel the words had touched him at very deep and revealing level. It had stripped him of everything he felt protected him, and paved the way to exposing his vulnerability. Suddenly, he leaned in toward me. The expression on his face suggested there was something he still wanted to tell me. It was as if he'd lost all touch with God and the world around him, and he wanted so desperately to get it back. It was deeply embedded in his soul and was now begging to come out.

Our faces were now eye-to-eye, about six inches apart. There was an argument going on with two other inmates next to us, but Truman didn't flinch. Not once. He just sat right there on the edge of his bunk, staring at me, and said in a solemn tone, "Preach, your words remind me of my preacher down back home, way back when I was growing up."

I somehow think I knew what he meant by that. I could have quoted him anything from the Bible, but it wasn't just the words off the paper. It was also the love, tears, and compassion shown to him that really touched him. I'm sure of it. Ever since my near-death experience, something in me had profoundly changed. The visions I was seeing were now helping to change some of the inmates' lives, and at times I could feel their pain deeply, like an empath.

"I've killed in Iraq and all over, and if you ain't the real deal, I'll snap yo' neck! I'll kill you! Don't play with me, man! You hear me? Don't play with me like that! I ain't never had no problem killing people. It's all the same to me!" he yelled.

He had finally released what was plaguing his spirit after all these years. His body was now trembling. Behind the vacant look in his eyes it seemed he was reliving snapshots of every person he'd ever killed in war. It was disturbing and sad.

"Back there at that God-awful place, they made me a cold-blooded killer, and now I can't turn it off in my head! You hear me, Preach?" he shouted in anguish. "I can't turn it off!"

He had the look in his eyes like he'd seen so much death; it caused his face to grimace in despair. He sat there with his eyes fixed on mine and his hand twitching like it was holding the trigger of a loaded AK-47. These were the tragic symptoms of post-traumatic stress syndrome (PTSD).

"I get real serious when it comes to God!" he said. "I had given up on Him. I'd lost my way, but now I need to hear those kinds of words and see those real tears—other than mine—of someone caring again. It's showing me I can be freed from all that death that surrounded me. Preach, it makes them kinda words more real, man. They really got to me! I don't wanna be waking up in the middle of the night with them kinda dreams no mo'. I just can't take it."

The tears continued to stream down his coal-dark face. It was as if a glass of hot water had just been spilled on that lacquer piano, and no one had ever cared enough to dry it off. What I had just witnessed was that intense. Truman tried to fight it off, but the more he did, the harder the tears flowed. His head slowly dropped down from the unbearable weight of his broken spirit. I held him like a father holding a newborn child.

His face was now swollen with rage, yet he looked freed from whatever had been troubling his spirit—if only for that moment. Once again, it was that inner child who had been neglected for so long. The next thing I knew, I found my eyes welling up for him again. I was that moved by his display of raw emotion. I wanted to show him he wasn't alone.

He raised his head and said to me, "Preach, my brother, I'll follow you around this whole damn earth to hear you bring comforting words like that! The Holy Spirit touched something in me, man," he cried.

Without another word spoken, he lay back on his bunk in contentment, put his hands behind his head, and stared at the ceiling until he fell asleep.

I opened my Bible and read a few powerful Scriptures from the book of Matthew; how Jesus spoke about having compassion for others. The dorm was now quiet and the lights were dim. I wrapped a blanket around my shoulders to stave off the freezing-cold air in the room. An inmate came over shivering and asked if I had an extra one. I handed him one, then sat there and meditated, praying for Truman for hours. I truly felt for him. I knew he would be transferring soon because something deep in my soul told me our work together was done.

At about two o'clock in the morning, the sound of the guard calling out bunk numbers came over the loudspeakers. You could hear the rustling of inmates waking up. "Roll it up for transfer!" the guard instructed. This time, Truman's number was called. I woke him up to tell him the sad news. Tears came down his face again as he slowly got up to pack his belongings. I told him it was too bad our time had been cut short. I hugged him and we said our goodbyes.

"That's how God works," I told him.

He said he would take the experience with him and never forget it; he told me how moved he was by the words of compassion. Once again, I'd been sent another troubled soul to bring God's words of comfort. I was so grateful for the experience of seeing Him at work amongst those who'd been broken. Knowing I'd been there myself is why it made me so emotional to talk to them. I understood it all too well. Within minutes Truman was hidden amongst the crowd of inmates who were being transferred with him.

As the metallic sound of the door unlocked to let them out, that was the last time I saw him. This time, it sounded different. Maybe it was reminding me of the sound of the latch on a birdcage being unlocked, and Truman was the bird finally being let out spiritually to fly to unknown heights.

God bless you, Truman, my brother, who fought for our country. Stay forever strong in the Spirit.

Just Another Court Date

"Just send me back to county jail."

Those were the words said after I stood up calmly and addressed Ronnie, my public defender, from the opposite side of a cold glass cubicle. We were in the attorneys' cell that day. It was a small cell located on the Criminal Courts floor in San Fernando.

"I won't settle for a plea bargain!" I told him as he leaned back in his chair to listen.

Ronnie was twirling a pen in his mouth. He removed it and started playing a rhythmic cadence on the table.

"Why can't you get that?" I asked him to no avail.

"As your attorney, I think you need to focus on trying to settle and get out of this dangerous place. It's filled with psychopaths and murders," he said convincingly.

Meanwhile, a group of gang member onlookers stared at him and me in sheer disbelief at the difference in conversations taking place in the room. It was a contrast to the commotion of more serious and violent cases being discussed in the cell. The atmosphere was chaotic.

"If they're offering me forty instead of life, I'll take it!" shouted an inmate to his attorney. He seemed content with the offer just made to him.

They were handing out long conviction sentences faster than trick-or-treaters getting candy on

Halloween, I thought. It was sad. There was no privacy for any of the inmates, unfortunately, as we continued frantically trying to take advantage of the short time allotted with our attorneys. This was all before heading into the courtroom to face the judge. Most were scared, even though they tried to hide it. How could you not be? It was obvious that most of us had public defenders for counsel, yet we knew that things would be much better if we had a paid attorney willing to fight harder for our cases.

Another inmate yelled at his attorney in disgust as he tried to get his bail reduced from two million dollars to a half million for a double homicide. Ronnie and I paused to listen.

"Get back in there and work your magic!" the inmate told him. "Don't make me have to come on the other side of this glass, you hear me, fool?" he roared, clearly frustrated with the news.

Ronnie and his colleague exchanged looks of frustration and disgust with the irate inmate. Clearly they both felt their work wasn't appreciated, even by me, for that matter.

"Ronnie, I've told you this before. Nothing has changed since my last court date here with you, and I'll say it to you again: I'm innocent! It's unfortunate this poor lady has made false allegations against me far above and beyond what really happened that night. I can only imagine how frightened she and her son were, but still, the truth is the truth, and this is far from it. This has to be a misdemeanor at best. I'm still confident it is God who will ultimately decide my fate here, not the judge, not her, and—no disrespect—not even you. I wish I could take that night back. Maybe one day, if she's open, I'd be willing to apologize to her in person," I told him.

"I doubt that would ever happen," he said.

You could hear the weary passion in my voice. I was determined not to let the system break me like it had done to so many others who were institutionalized around me.

"Really?" Ronnie said. "It doesn't make a lot of sense what you're trying to take on here. This is real life we're dealing with here, Mr. Palmer, in case you didn't know it. You can't save people. This isn't some kind of fantasy movie you seem to have going on inside your head," he responded.

Ronnie got up and walked out the conference cell. He paused for a moment, turned around, and said, "As your attorney, I'm advising you to settle this case quickly and take the felony strike along with the three-year probation the judge is offering you and walk today. I've been doing this for a while now, and judging by the evidence in your preliminary hearing, you might want to think about it more seriously."

He put me in complete shock after he finished explaining how the system worked. I felt let down by it and by him.

"I would be willing to serve the maximum time of four years given here before I'll give a guilty plea," I told him. "Go in there and tell the judge that for me."

"I think you may want to calm down. I don't think you know what you're saying. I think it's a great deal he's offering and probably your only deal," Ronnie said with a stern look on his face.

He turned around to leave the small room. He was incensed and frustrated with me as the door slammed shut behind him, leaving me in utter shock and dismay.

"Hey, homie, are you crazy, my man? You'd better take that deal they're offering you. It doesn't get much better than that in here," said a Southsider who'd come over to me.

I asked him how much time he was facing.

"Double life, homie; double life," he said as he slapped five to another gang inmate.

They started to laugh hysterically, flashing synchronized gang signs to each other. I appreciated his concern but I was sticking to my plan of not capitulating to the system, because I was innocent. It's much more of an uphill challenge when the system says you're guilty until proven innocent.

What came to my mind—especially after hearing all that—was, 'Am I crazy, or am I truly following my God's word? And my attorney's words: "This is real life we're dealing with here."

I just wasn't sure any more if I was grasping it. Only time would tell about the uncertainty in the decision I'd just made. The guard's voice instructed us to wrap it up with our attorneys. They cuffed us and led us back to the holding tanks on the floor below to wait for the bus to return us to L.A. County Jail.

I'd learned that every inmate in prison is not a criminal, contrary to popular belief. It is the very antithesis of that understanding. The California judicial system is set up so that if you are innocent, you can still wind up having to plea bargain your way out, which sometimes means accepting a long prison sentence. I lost count of how many inmates I had prayed to stay strong. There are a lot of good people caught up in a broken system and it's time for reform, but there are quite a few who do belong there. They are without a conscience and wouldn't hesitate to kill you in a minute.

Most inmates who were awaiting trial told me they were aware of their public defenders' ineptitude. This made them feel that their freedom wasn't worth fighting for any more, especially when they already knew the outcome. They had given up hope for fairness in the penal system. At that moment, the door opened and a female sheriff stood in the doorway and began calling off names.

"Jackson! Walker! Palmer! Corden! And Winston! Line it up!

We lined up single file for the ride back to the L.A. County Jail.

"Anybody got a ticket for belongings?" the other guard asked. "Surrender it if you want your sh*t back!" He told us to step up the line if we wanted to make the bus waiting outside to get us back to County on time.

We then prepared to board the bus. The guard chained me to two other black inmates (one was a gang member), and we stepped into the line to wait to board.

"Don't get on the bus until I tell you to!" he yelled as another guard escorted a chain of high-powered Latino Southsiders onto the bus first. They put them into individual cages, separating them from us and the general population. They were the most serious of the alleged offenders. 'K2' is what they called them, 'keep-aways', because they couldn't get along with the general jail population. K2s could be any race; in this case, they were Mexican.

"Okay, whites next!" he shouted.

They boarded, separating them from the Southsiders and us. He sent them to the rear cages. Some of those men were members of the most-serious gangs in the country, like the Aryan Skinheads. One had a tattoo on his head that read, "I hate Jews!" We boarded last, when he gave us the signal once the others were all contained in their sections.

"Blacks next!"

Mostly Bloods gang members were in my group, some just as dangerous as the other gangs. We noticed there were girls on this trip, which caused the Latino inmates in the back cages to start whistling.

"How long has it been since you've seen something like these?" a short-haired, tattooed, Latino girl yelled out as she flashed her breasts to the Southsiders.

I noticed the sound of the buses pulling off as the guard turned on the radio and air, and we headed back across town. Listening to Tupac on the ride back, I was lost in a daze. I stared out at the California sun. It greeted my skin. It had been a month—my last court date—since I'd felt the sun's caressing rays or seen the outside. During bus rides, back and forth from court were the only times I saw it.

I laughed, thinking about how mesmerized the Southsiders were by the female inmate's breasts. From the conversations I'd heard, it had been years since some of them had touched or had any contact with a woman. Sadly for some, it might never happen again in their lifetime, especially those who were waiting to start long-term sentences—some life, and even death row. Those were the kind of inmates who were on that bus trip back.

'Lord, help us all,' I thought. I bowed my head in silent prayer for the inmates and their alleged victims, knowing everyone can receive God's forgiveness if we'll just ask for it. It was, after all, just another court date.

The Approval

I can clearly remember and will never forget the day I met Antonio Ramirez. I'd just returned from court, and the jail dorm was bustling with returnees, like myself. There was always a large inmate changeover on the days we came back from court. Some arrived who had just been arrested. Some were awaiting trial to be sentenced and moved to a prison to serve their time— for some, maybe life. While putting my court papers away at the head of my bunk, I could hear a familiar voice standing behind me. It was Luis, the leader of the Latino Southsiders gang. We had become friends through the prayer work I was doing for some of the gangs, and because of it, he was a big supporter.

"Hey, Preach. I gotta homie here I wanna introduce you to. He's been preaching in other jail dorms to inmates like yourself. I told him about you. I think you guys will hit it off well."

"Preach, right? I'm Antonio Ramirez. Just call me Tony. My homie here says some of the inmates come to you to hear about God and learn meditation. It can help some of them to clear their minds of this horrible place, I'd imagine. You lead most of the prayer groups for all the inmates and gangs in here, right?"

I told him I did. He then went on to say he was doing the same in other jail dorms before he'd come there.

"I'm just trying to bring God's love to some of the inmates. Maybe it's time for all of us to start thinking about changing our lives, right?" I responded.

He said that was why he'd turned his life over to Him. "I'm facing life without parole or maybe the death penalty."

"I'm so sorry to hear that, Tony. It's my pleasure to meet you as well. Maybe we can do some work here together?"

"Yeah, I would like that."

Over those next few days, I loved the work I did with Tony. He had a genuinely kind spirit and loved God. I remember telling him one night that he was the first person I'd met in my entire life in whose face I actually believed I saw redemption. It was striking. He was very humbled, and that's when he shared his thoughts with me.

"Preach, you wanna know what one of my greatest wishes in life is? It's for God to give me some sort of sign, a sign that he approves of the work I'm doing with the inmates."

I thought it was an interesting request. Here was a man at a crucial crossroads of his life—he was facing life or death in prison—yet he was still doing God's work. What a true dedication. When we got together I tried to convince Tony that I felt God had to be very proud of him, and that I knew he'd asked Him for forgiveness a thousand times over for whatever it was that brought him here. I prayed on it that night for him.

Tony was a true beacon of light to me. His aura was so amazing and his knowledge of the Word was extensive. We did a lot of praying together; he was a fierce prayer warrior. During that time, if an inmate was troubled we went into deep prayer for them together. We held all-night prayer vigils. He was awesome. But despite all of that, whenever we were done praying with the inmates for the night, he always ended by telling me about his wish. I really felt for him. I was beginning to see how much it meant to him. Tony's bunk was just across from mine, and most of the time we read our Bibles together until the lights became so dim we would have to stop for the night.

This night was no different from any other. We were done and I walked over to my bunk to do my meditation before turning in. There Tony was, trying to squeeze in the last few minutes of reading before the lights when totally dark. I started meditating, and within a few minutes, God reminded me of a vision He'd shown me of the black Catholic saint, St. Martin de Porres, while meditating that day on November 3, 2011, which was also the same date of St. Martin's death. Now He was bringing it back to my memory.

Since the night of that incident I hadn't told anyone about it, except my sister Gloria. The fact that St. Martin had died at the age of fifty-nine made it even clearer because I was now fifty-nine. I now saw the connections. He said Tony wanted to know if He approved of what he was doing with his work for Him, but didn't have a way of knowing. He told me to go over to Tony and ask him who St. Martin de Porres was. In that moment, he would know that only God could have known that, letting him know that He approved of his work. I wasn't sure if I was talking to myself at that moment; it was just too unbelievable! He had spoken to me many times, but this was different. It was a big question Tony wanted answered.

I followed the instructions and got up and walked over to him as he was just getting ready to turn in. "Tony, you got a minute? I want to ask you a question."

"Sure, Preach. What is it?"

"Well, I'm not quite sure how to put it. I know you've told me you've asked God if He approves of the job you're doing. I was on my bunk meditating, and He came to me and reminded me of a vision He showed me years ago. At that time, I wasn't sure why I saw that vision, but after all these years, that answer came just a few minutes ago from Him. So, when I ask you who was the person in that vision, God said you would know. This will be the sign you seek from Him, telling you that you are doing a good job."

Tony was so excited to find out what I was talking about, but after telling him, I knew he thought I was crazy. I had no clue what was going to happen. I took a deep breath and said, "His name is St. Martin de Porres."

Tony was so stunned, he dropped to his knees shaking, with tears filling his eyes. "Oh my God, Preach! That's just not possible for you to know St. Martin de Porres is my patron saint! He was given to me as a kid, and still is to this very day! This is truly a miracle that God has given me a sign through you! It's just truly unbelievable, my friend."

Tony just stood there in amazement at the news. I was still in shock myself. Until then I'd had no idea that this was the reason why I'd seen St. Martin de Porres. The look in his eyes told me he needed time with God right now. That was a lot for both of us to take in. I'd actually just witnessed God giving one of his faithful servants a priceless gift through a sign. Who on this earth can say that?

I finished my meditation and I told God that what He'd done for Tony was truly an amazing moment I'd witnessed. I guess acceptance is everything to most of us in this world. I just can't imagine what that felt like for him. He'd said it would mean everything to him. I slowly drifted off to sleep after that. My spirit had been filled.

The next morning I had to get up at three o'clock for court. I noticed Tony was still asleep when I walked past him. Contentment was still written all over his face. I still couldn't imagine what it had been like for him to get a sign from God that night.

I was at court most of that day, but when I returned, an inmate walked up to me and handed me a piece of paper. It was from Tony. It read: *God bless you. Stay strong in our work. It has been a pleasure. Anthony Ramirez.*

I immediately felt sad because I hadn't gotten a chance to say goodbye before he'd left. In jail, you never know how long someone will stay will one place. So, you learn to take advantage of the time spent with an inmate you really get along with. Tony was one of those inmates I had a great respect for. I'd enjoyed every minute of what we had accomplished together. In those few days, I had a chance to meet an amazing man, who showed me firsthand what the power of God's grace, forgiveness, and redemption can do to one's soul. God wanted Tony to know that his transformation was noteworthy. He was very proud of the man he'd become, despite the one he may have been (I had never asked him – that's something you just don't do in jail/prison). What I did know was he'd given his life over to Him in servitude and He'd rewarded him for it. I later found out that Tony had been given life without parole.

Anthony Ramirez, you are a soul on this road of life whom I will always remember. Thank you, my friend, for your generous spiritual strength and wisdom. Wherever you are, I know inmates' lives will be forever changed by your presence.

RICARDO'S STORY

I had now been incarcerated in the dangerous part of the L.A. County Jail for six months. Despite those constant dangers around me I was still meditating seven hours a day, seven days a week. I was becoming more spiritually enlightened, and my relationship with God at this point was further being enriched and deeply rewarded from the prayer work I was doing with the hundreds of inmates I'd met from different gangs.

During those meditation periods I had conversations with Him daily, and what I learned taught me how to let my spirit become like water, to constantly allow it to be cleansed from the darkness of jail life. After each meditation period, I grew closer to understanding the purpose of living in continuous servitude. There was a burning inside me like that of an eternal raging fire. I was becoming one with God's Spirit, receiving the pure incarnation of His love for myself. Sharing it with the inmates around me was like the first breath of a newborn child and the welcome tears that stream from a mother's eyes.

Later that day, after my meditation, it was now time for my prayer group with the inmates. There were constantly new faces, and on this particular day, I noticed someone who I'd seen around the jail but had never come to the group before. I asked him to stand up and introduce himself to the group.

"My name is Ricardo."

One of the first things I would do when a new inmate (who was usually a gang member) joined the group was have him introduce himself, then bless his rivals and their families. In this case, Ricardo said he wasn't in a gang. He was in jail for being constantly arrested for possession of crystal meth.

It was usually standing-room-only, because the Spyder tables in the day room only sat four. I would normally have a closed Bible in my hand. Sometimes, when an inmate would ask me to turn to a particular Scripture, I would drop it on the table and, miraculously, it would open to the page with that specific Scripture. It would astound the inmates every time it happened, including myself. I always told them it was God's way of saying He was there in that moment and was listening to their problems. After that, I would read the Word from the place where the Bible had opened, and offer prayer at the end for them and their loved ones on the outside.

When I finished that night and all the inmates had gone back to their bunks, Ricardo was still standing there. He looked as if he'd seen a ghost.

"How'd you do that?" he asked, still looking confused.

I told him it wasn't a magic trick, and if that was what he was looking for, one of the inmates over in the corner did great card tricks. "This is God communicating with the inmates, letting them know He hears them when that happens. A few of them get choked up when they hear that. A lot of them have told me they've never felt God's love before. That's what they say has made a lot of them criminals, and some even murderers. I'm only a messenger here to pray with them."

Ricardo apologized and said he wanted to learn how to do it for a personal reason that was dear to him. He told me his father was a wealthy land owner in Mexico. He had five sisters and he was the only son. His family knew he was a drug addict, always in and out of jail, and they felt he was a disgrace to the family name. His father was getting up in years and couldn't trust leaving him in charge of his fortune. He felt he would squander it on drugs. His mother said he was a son without a God. I could tell this was hurting him deeply as he struggled to get through the last part of his story.

"So, now Preach, let me tell you why I need to learn what you did today and what others here have told me they've witnessed on many other occasions. Because, if I tell my family about this man in here who says he's a messenger from God, maybe my mother will feel her prayers have been answered. If I tell them what I saw you do, and you taught me how, hopefully she will truly believe I have been touched by His Spirit."

In that moment, I knew in my heart that once again God had sent me another broken one, as I myself had once been.

"Ricardo, yes, I would be honored to guide you to His Spirit. I want you to come to me every afternoon after you see me finish my midday meditation. Oh yeah, don't forget to bring your Bible, okay?"

He said he didn't have one, so I gave him a brand-new, shiny, cobalt-colored one. He then walked away with a smile of contentment.

The next day after my midday meditation, Ricardo was standing there on time, Bible in hand. I could instantly tell by the fresh bends on the binding that he'd opened it that night in his bunk.

"Good afternoon, Preach; I'm ready. I spoke to my mom this morning and she said God is finally answering her prayers. She wants you to pray for our family."

I told him I would and asked, "You ready to get started?"

We spent hours that day with me teaching him how to meditate to first clear his mind. He was a great student.

In those next few days after the prayer group, Ricardo would always stay behind afterward. I was so proud of what he was trying to accomplish for his family, but even more importantly, I was happy for the relationship he was developing with God. The first thing he'd always say was, "Preach, again you opened the Bible right on those chapters. Am I getting close?"

I told him, "It isn't about how close or far you are; God's spirit is not a measurement. It's a receivership of your belief. When you truly believe in your spirit that it is real, that's when what is already there will appear in front of you, and in that moment, miracles will happen."

It had now been several weeks since we'd started, and on this particular day I could tell Ricardo's spirit was beginning to wane and get weary. He wasn't that perky, excited person when he'd first come to me. Because of that, I knew this was going to be his day.

"Ricardo, before you speak, I want you to follow exactly what I tell you, okay?"

He looked very puzzled, but was accommodating. I led him to the chair and he sat down. I instructed him to close his Bible and put it to the left of him, out of sight. I took his hands and asked him to close his eyes; then I said a prayer. I prayed "for the stream of his lost spirit to merge into the ocean of God's boundless love." Then I instructed him to not talk or open his eyes.

"Ricardo, reach to your left, stick your thumb in your closed Bible, and turn to Psalm 1:1." He did as he was instructed. "Now, open your eyes and see how much God loves you and that He hears your family's prayers."

"Oh my god! It's on Psalm 1:1!" Ricardo shouted. His head dropped on the table and he was sobbing like a child. "Preach, now I can tell my father what happened here today, and that I will never do drugs again in my life. I want him to be proud of me. I've received God in my life, and this was my proof."

I told him, "It isn't the size of the miracle; it's how big the source who sent it is."

Ricardo ran over to the phone to call his mother and tell her the news. When he came back, he said she couldn't wait to tell the rest of the family they'd received a sign from God for their son and family.

After that day, Ricardo continued doing his meditations with me and came to every prayer group for the remainder of his time there. He was soon released, and on the day he left, he told me he'd made a vow to God that he would keep Him in his life forever. His father couldn't wait for him to come to Mexico so he could embrace what he called "his Prodigal Son."

I never saw Ricardo again after that day, but I knew that what he'd received with his Bible would only become even greater and would comfort him in times of doubt throughout his journey.

The lights in the jail dorm were starting to lower for the night and inmates were preparing for sleep. I climbed up on my bunk and took a few minutes to meditate, to listen to the voice of God's Spirit saying, "The journey of a lost spirit is very long, but to find Me happens only in one's moment of realization that they were never lost." I thanked Him for His continued conversations of wisdom. I said a prayer, pulled the blanket up over me to stave off the cold air coming through the overhead vents, then went to sleep for the night. Despite being in jail, it had been another great day.

A QUICK DECISION

Some things in jail just couldn't be avoided at times, and fighting was one of them. I usually tried to break them up before they escalated into the dark zone, that area of no-return. Long incarcerations and solitary can do terrible things to a man's mind. It was always frightening jumping between two men three times your size who had nothing left in them to lose, who only had a pure disdain for each other. It was clearly a life-threatening challenge to take on.

I was adjusting to the new dorm when I ran into an inmate named Lewis. We were the only two who had been transferred together from our 9400 dorms just a few days ago. I knew I had seen him at the 9400 dorm, reading his Bible religiously every day. That, dominoes, and cards was how he served his time. His skin was medium brown, and he was quiet and very small-framed. Certain areas of his short hair had tufts of gray that resembled billowing clouds. He looked to be around my age—in his late fifties. As he was the only one I knew from the group, we immediately struck up a conversation and a friendship.

Lewis told me he couldn't read. He said the only book he could read was the Bible. I thought that was fascinating, and I would later write letters for him. He wasn't the only inmate who couldn't read any book but the Bible. Then you had those on the opposite end of the spectrum who were scholar equivalents, absolute geniuses in their own respect.

On this day, it started out as a typical one. Guys were working out on the makeshift gym bars attached under the staircase. Others were playing cards, while some were playing dominoes. The smell of pork rinds, hot pickles, pruno (jail liquor made by the inmates), and disgusting jail food, along with the putrid stench of the open bathroom facilities permeated the dorm area as mildew leaked from the dilapidated ceiling. There was the sound of toilets flushing from guys washing their clothes in it. Me? I was meditating on my bunk.

Out of those daily routines, my focus was suddenly shifted to the game of dominoes that had quickly escalated to the point of unbridled pride, which is dangerous in jail. At first I couldn't quite make out who it was because they were on the bottom level of the dorm, but it was only a matter of minutes before I saw them ascend the staircase to the second-level tier where I was situated. It was Lewis and his bunkmate Fred. Fred was what I called a gargantuan. He wasn't that tall but he was wide. He worked out every day, all day. That was his routine. He could lift anything and anybody, so you didn't want to piss him off as Lewis obviously had just done, over something so trivial.

"I don't want you as a bunkmate anymore!" Fred yelled at Lewis.

"You're kidding me, right? All I did was beat you at a game of dominoes," Lewis said with a perplexed look.

Fred walked over to their bunk, grabbed Lewis' mattress off the bottom, and slung it across the room.

We—the onlookers—were stunned. In jail, you just don't touch another man's belongings. Lewis walked over to pick up his mattress, and that's when Fred grabbed him from behind in a chokehold of death. Lewis' small frame didn't stand a chance. Fred was choking him with everything he had, and that was a lot. After a few minutes, Lewis went limp. His eyes were closed and he wasn't moving. His face was bruised.

Quickly, I jumped down from my bunk, ran over to them, and looked at Lewis' face. He wasn't responding. Fred was so muscular, he dwarfed Lewis like the shadow of a skyscraper over a tricycle. He now had veins protruding from his neck. That's how hard he was choking him. I ran behind Fred, took a deep breath and grabbed him from behind. Again, in jail, that was something you just didn't do—come from behind another man or touch him, let alone grab him with everything you had. I stretched my arms as wide as I could and still couldn't fully grab him. Fred was huge and his back was as hard as the concrete floor, which my face was about to meet if he turned around.

I was now treading in a very dangerous area. If Fred let go of Lewis and grabbed me, he would surely kill me or beat me down pretty bad, and I knew it. But something in me was willing to take that chance. Sometimes you have to do what must be done without concern for your own life in order to save another. I had learned this the hard way, breaking up fights almost every week. The harder Fred choked Lewis, the tighter I grabbed him. I knew something would have to give soon. Suddenly, he let him go. Lewis' limp body dropped. He was gone.

Fred, as I figured, came straight for me. He was shouting every obscenity that entered his head. The cold chill off his nose touched mine, and as he cursed, his spit was hitting my face like rain. I retained my composure in spite of his tirade. I didn't budge one inch from him. Was I scared? No. In that moment, I began to pray for the darkness that had taken over his spirit to be lifted, so he could maybe see the light. I was concerned about Lewis lying over there on the ground, his body lifeless. I knew God would protect me and give me the strength I needed—not physically, but spiritually—to stand up to this out-of-control inmate.

At that moment, I looked over. Lewis had regained consciousness and was gagging, trying to catch his breath. Whew! I exhaled. He was all right for now, but he wasn't out of the woods just yet. What if Fred wasn't finished? Judging by the look on his face, it looked like he wasn't. I then did something I knew would shock Fred so he wouldn't go back and finish. I jumped up on my bunk right in front of him, sat in a meditating position, closed my eyes, and began to pray again. I sat there wondering if he would drag me off and kill me, but I fought the fear and kept praying. The entire dorm was dead quiet at this point, waiting for him to grab me.

Suddenly, someone was tapping on my mattress. I opened my eyes and it was Fred. His eyes had the look of remorse. He looked at me and just two words came out of his mouth. They were simply, "Thank you." I pointed a finger in the air and told him God had already forgiven him.

At this point, the sheriffs came running up the stairs and grabbed him. They had watched the entire thing as it happened. They took Fred away to the hole. He was facing add-charges, which meant he could be tried for assault or attempted murder. That could possibly add years to his sentence, and if he had killed Lewis, it could have added a life sentence.

I went over to Lewis to see if he was okay. He was wheezing and gagging, and still trying to catch his breath. Fred had almost killed him, he knew, and if God hadn't given me the strength in that moment he would have been dead that day. He thanked me with everything he had left. I helped him over to his bunk to sit down.

"I'm pressing charges, Preach!" he fumed when he had caught his breath.

The sheriff came up and gave Lewis a form to fill out. He was livid. Nobody could blame him, especially when Fred really had tried to kill him. It was then that God gave me the words to tell Lewis. I asked him what he thought Fred was thinking about as he sat in the hole. Lewis said he didn't care and asked why he should be concerned about Fred.

"Lewis, you believe in God, right?"

He nodded his head yes. I asked him if he wondered if Fred believed as well. Once again he said he didn't care as he filled out the forms to charge him. I then told him that his own belief in God had put me there at the right time to save his life.

"I would be willing to bet you Fred is sitting in the hole as we speak, hopefully praying to his God, which is the same as yours," I told him. "Doesn't he deserve a blessing if he's praying right now? Lewis, you now hold the power within your pen to spare him from add-charges. Let God bless him for his mistake." I told Lewis he should have seen Fred's face when he tapped my mattress to tell me "thank you" for saving him from making a huge mistake.

"Lewis, let him get his blessing," I begged him again as he finished up the last details on the form.

I could see the sheriffs waiting at the foot of the stairs for him to bring it down to them. "Don't do it, my brother," I begged him again.

He looked at me then looked at the form. "That fool almost killed me!" he shouted, heading for the stairs with the form in his hand. I stood there and closed my eyes, praying he wouldn't do it. He got to the stairs, and just as he was getting ready to walk down, he suddenly turned, walked over to me, and tore it up.

"You're right, Preach, he deserves a blessing too."

Lewis went down to the sheriffs and let them know he'd changed his mind. They turned around and left. I could tell he felt good about the decision he'd just made. He'd held the power to bless someone and he'd chosen wisely, using compassion just as Jesus would have. I told him it took a real man of prayer to do what he had just done. He thanked me again for saving his life. I told him God was the one he should be thanking. Give Him the glory; I was just a messenger sent by Him.

As inmates were coming in from court, Lewis ran over and told everyone his story of how God had saved his life. He was truly grateful.

Always A Gladiator

After we left the courtroom that day, my attorney again tried convincing me to take the deal that had been offered. Once again, I told him no way, and it was another stalemate. I wanted to go to trial, whether I won or lost. If I lost I would be facing a possible four-year sentence in a penitentiary. I wasn't budging, nor was the prosecutor. If it meant me getting four years, I would just continue God's work there. I told my attorney there was no way I'd lose either way. The judge was holding firm in giving me a felony strike. There was no way I was going to leave that place with three years' probation and a felony strike for something I simply did not do. They knew it was a misdemeanor at best. I didn't care about the consequences. My faith was now at its strongest.

I was very frustrated and wanted to go back to county jail to finish God's work. The judge made it clear I could have walked if I had been willing to take his deal. I had made the tough decision to stay in county jail and ignore my trial. I prayed on it and now it was in God's hands. I had officially released myself spiritually from the burden of it once again. The only thing on my mind was servitude to the inmates. I felt in my heart I could make a difference. I was now more committed than ever.

I would rather stay in jail and preach to the inmates like I was doing. It was God's work that mattered to me, not the crooked judicial system that I'd witnessed since being incarcerated. It was sad how their only concern was the convictions on record. It had nothing to do with whether you were innocent or not. Judges and other officials wanted high conviction rates on their record for re-elections.

It was getting late in the evening in the dorm. I was sitting on my bunk in the lotus position, doing my usual meditation. The inmates had just finished chow. You could tell by the smell in the air of the mystery meats floating in fat they served us most of the time. It wasn't palatable. Inmates often voiced their opinion to the trustees, but they usually fell on deaf ears.

A few minutes later, my meditation was interrupted by what sounded like an argument between two rival gang members. Within minutes, it had turned into a full-on argument. I continued to meditate and not let it bother me as it escalated. I knew at any minute a fight would break out. I abhor violence. I tried to ignore it. The entire dorm knew I was against it, especially as I was there trying to do God's work, and most of them respected it. They were used to me breaking up the fights no matter how bad they were.

Judging by the tone of their voices, this one seemed to be getting closer to my bunk. After a while, you knew just when a fight would erupt. Was I becoming institutionalized like so many others there? I opened my eyes to a sight I dreaded.

They were now fighting and there was blood everywhere. I had become acquainted with both men just weeks ago. John was about 260 pounds and medium height. Eric was about 250 pounds and six-foot-two. Both of them were big, muscular guys. They were fighting their way around the dorm. By the time they got to my side, John was a bloody mess. It was pouring from his head and face. I knew it was only minutes before he would be in the danger zone. The crowd of inmates was following close behind, egging them on. They were now right in front of my bunk. I knew it had to be stopped.

So here I was, wondering if I should risk myself once again to try to bring order back to the dorm. They were beating each other to death and it was brutal. Eric was definitely getting the best of John as I watched from my bunk. It had gone on long enough and nobody was interested in stopping them. It was a blood sport for some; they were gladiators. That's just how it was in jail. For most it broke the monotony from the boring and mundane life of incarceration. After months of being in there, I was beginning to see the picture. I just wanted to do the right thing before one of them got seriously hurt.

I jumped down from my bunk and stepped between them. That was very risky, especially with gang members. They usually fought for keeps. It was not a game of two guys playing around. They were trying to kill each other, and they were twice my size. They could have turned on me at any minute. Who was I to get in the middle of someone's beef against another inmate?

Once again somehow, the power of the Spirit was in control as I looked them both straight in the eye, extending my arms between them to stop. I asked both of them if they trusted me. After a minute or so, they both nodded. I couldn't show signs of fear; that would have proven fatal. They both, individually, at one time or another, had come to me for prayer. I then asked them "In the Name of God" to please go back to their respective bunks and cool off. They did as I asked. The crowd of inmates was shocked. I believe they were starting to believe God was real. An older inmate as I couldn't possibly have done it every time himself. Soon they began to disperse.

A few minutes later, I walked over to Eric's bunk, holding two bags of precious potato chips, which are like gold in jail. I asked him if he still trusted God. He said yes. I asked him to come with me. Everyone in the dorm thought I was crazy when they saw me lead Eric over to John's bunk on the other side of the room, knowing they hadn't cooled off yet. When we reached John's bunk I asked him if he trusted God as well. He also said yes. I then took both of their hands and put a bag of chips in them. I took their other hands and made them shake them. Minutes later, they were walking through the dorm, hugging each other like best friends.

The only thing that came to my mind that night was, 'God, You are truly amazing! None of this would be possible without Your love for us all in here.'

A Braided Cross, Part 1

I had spoken to my mom and sister the night before. They were in great spirits, but today was another court day, which usually meant getting up by three in the morning, having breakfast, then walking in single-file, accompanied by armed guards to the 'tank.' The tank is in the jail, where you wait for your bus to take you to court at around seven. I sat there waiting in the segregated tank, which was packed to the brim. There was always that permeating and disgusting smell of dried urine. It was to remind you that you were in L.A. County Jail, in case you forgot.

Inmates were bragging about who was going to get the longest sentences.

"I'm facing sixty years, Johnny. How about you?"

"I got you beat, dog! I'm facing a life sentence. Let me see you beat that!"

It would usually continue with the false bravado until the buses arrived. I felt deeply for these lost young men who believed getting a life sentence was something to brag about. They couldn't be more than twenty years old. A life just starting, now wasted. What about their families and the poor victims? If these men were found guilty, was there any remorse? These young men were just some of the challenges I was given to preach to. Bring them all to God, and try to save the ones who hadn't gotten to this point yet.

There is an endless revolving door of recidivism for these young men of all colors, but mainly men of color.

Most were attached at the hip to their gangs. I usually tried to spend more time with these young types. I had to fight my spirit to sometimes not get frustrated and just let God continue doing His work through me; I continued to pray for and with them.

The bus finally arrived and we boarded. We were usually chained to another inmate you'd probably never see again in your life. When we arrived, I met with the judge to discuss my case. I told him nothing had changed and I still wanted to move forward with the trial. I knew the charges were trumped up and I was innocent. I was willing to prove that, no matter what it took. I had to be a man of my own convictions otherwise what else did I stand for? This meant a quick, five-minute decision for the judge. All he had to do was set a date for some time in the future. Then it was time to make the trip back across town to L.A. County Jail.

For the trip back, we were chained again to somebody we'd probably never see again. Considering L.A. County Jail's population was somewhere over 19,000 at any given time, it made those odds even greater. On this day I was chained to a very young African American man. After we boarded the bus and sat down, we introduced ourselves.

"Hi. Inmates here call me, Preach. What's your name?"

"Nice to meet you. My name is Loren."

The jolt of the bus as it started its journey distracted us for a second as the driver turned on the radio. Loren went on to tell me he was only nineteen and had gotten arrested just that last week. He said he was out with friends who happened to be in a gang and someone had been killed. He was blamed for the incident and was now facing life. In that moment, his entire spirit dropped. I asked him if he believed in God. He said yes.

"Loren, let me pray for you, if you don't mind."

He said he didn't mind. After I prayed for him, he told me his family was pretty sad right now. He wanted to be a minister, but look what was possibly going to happen to his life. I saw he had a duffle bag sitting next to him. I asked him to take out his Bible and turn to a particular scripture.

"How did you know I had a Bible?" he asked.

When he took it out, I had him read it out loud over the sound of the music. That's when he looked at me and asked who I was.

"No way! How did you know that was my favorite scripture?"

"I didn't know. It was God Who did," I shared with him. "He knows your commitment to Him. He knows what's in your heart, whether you're innocent or guilty. He doesn't judge you if you come to Him for forgiveness, or strength in proving your innocence."

"Preach, what if I get a lot of years for something I didn't do? I really wanted to be an ordained preacher like yourself."

"Loren, I'm not an ordained preacher. It's just a name the inmates in here have given me because of the work I do. I'm only a faithful servant of God, which you can be as well. Let's say, if for some reason you do get convicted of the crime, just think about the amazing work Paul did while he was incarcerated. Most of his best work was from jail. God will decide your outcome, and if it's His will for you to be here, then make it count and do His great work as Paul chose to do.

"You see, Loren, it doesn't matter where we are when we do God's work. The main thing is to do it no matter the conditions we're faced with. I'm here and don't know for how long, but in the meantime, my faith says to bide that time serving and saving souls. In Him, *know that all things are working for my good.* We just need to learn how to trust that."

I took his hands and made him close his eyes so I could pray for the both of us. I prayed for us to stay strong in the Word and to continue to ask for the strength from God to preach it.

"So, Preach, now I think I get it. I can't wait to tell my family that, if for some reason I don't get out—I hope I'm not convicted—but if I am, maybe my calling will be to save souls from here with a ministry. That really calms my spirit. Thank you, my brother."

I could see a bit of relief break through his spirit, like the morning rays of the sun.

The bus had now pulled into the jail as the large fence opened to let it in.

"Preach, quick, before we get off. Here, take this cross I made from the string of my jail-assigned pants and shirt."

As he put it around my neck I told him I was honored to have it. I could see it was beautifully crafted. We got off the bus and merged with the other returning inmates. There were thousands—mostly gang members—all bustling to get back to their dorms. It was now time to head back to ours. I hugged Loren and told him to stay strong in the Word as I reminded him of the powerful words of Christ in Matthew 16:24: *"If any of you wants to be my follower, you must give up your own way, take up your cross, and follow me."*

The one he'd just given me could be symbolic of that for both of us. There was still a lot of hard work ahead, saving lost souls of inmates, and it was just beginning for that young man. I just knew he was going to do an amazing job preaching the Word, no matter where his journey would take him.

He yelled out before taking the elevator to his dorm, "Preach! Please don't ever forget me!"

"Don't worry, my brother, I won't."

I raised the cross he'd given me and kissed it. He disappeared into the crowd.

A Braided Cross, Part 2

Four months had passed since my encounter with Loren. I was now into my ninth month of incarceration and my spirit had gotten weary, but I was still determined to push on with my preaching to the inmates. I knew there would sometimes be days like this, but it was so important to continue God's valuable work that the inmates and I were so in need of: redemption, grace, forgiveness, salvation. All spiritual food for the edification and survival of the eternal soul.

I meditated for three hours, did my Bible study and prayer work, then got ready to start my day ministering with the inmates. As I prepared my papers, I was approached by a six-foot-four inmate who looked South American. He had stacks of large, bound books in his arms.

"Are you, Preach?" he asked.

I replied I was. I immediately noticed where he'd had a tattoo removed from his forehead. It was a cross.

"My name is Luis. I used to be a Believer," he said.

"He still believes in you."

"So, Preach, tell me why did they send me over to you? I'm facing life without parole for the alleged killing of a man. My public defender didn't share my same interests, so I decided to take on my own case. They let me go to the jail library to get the books I need."

When he said that, three jail dorm inmates who were enforcers walked up to us.

"Hey, crazy man, are you starting trouble again? They just kicked you out of the last dorm you were in."

"Don't make us have to throw your ass out of here this time for good! You know you ain't welcome around here."

"Six of us will stomp you out if you start up again, you hear me?"

Luis just shrugged it off and gave them a dark look. They warned him again and he finally said he would act right. I didn't know why they were so mad at him, but it must have been pretty bad. I could feel that Luis was definitely a wounded soul, and his spirit had become very dark because of it. That's why I knew God had sent him to me.

"I'm a troublemaker! That's what I like to do when you bother me! I can make your life miserable!" he warned.

He was staring at me without a smile or any emotion. I knew I needed to get his attention first before reading him the word of God. He was a 'doubting Thomas'. He was momentarily distracted by a quarterback on TV yelling out calls for a play. Then came the loud yells from inmates.

"Wow!"

"He missed it!"

That's when I asked him to listen to the voice of God and let Him calm his distressed spirit.

"Luis, do me a favor. Keep looking me straight in the eyes." I held up the cross Loren had given me four months previously. "Now, what if I told you, God is telling me right this minute that you are attached somehow to this braided cross?"

"I'd tell you that you and God are both crazy. That's what I'd tell you!"

I could tell he was getting very irritable, and the last thing the dorm needed was an out-of-control inmate they had already warned.

"Luis, God wants me to tell you a short story that only He would know how He has connected you to it. Hopefully, by showing you this, you will see it's no coincidence you're standing right here for me to preach to you about His Word, which can maybe offer you redemption and salvation for your soul..."

After I told Luis the story of how God had chained me to this young inmate on the bus ride back to jail and now I was standing there with a braided cross he'd given me, he asked, "So, why are you telling me this story? And why did God tell you this person has something to do with me? I still don't understand."

"Luis, God is never wrong. Ask me the young man's name and I'll prove it."

"Okay; what's his name?"

"His name is Loren."

"Oh my God! No way! That's not possible!" He broke down and started crying. Disbelief was written all over his face. "Preach, this is just not possible!"

He began to describe what he looked like and said, "This same inmate Loren was my cellmate over a year ago. There's over nineteen thousand inmates in here, and for him to be the one you're connecting that cross and myself to is amazing! God's got my attention," he said. He sat down, lowered his head, and continued shaking it in disbelief.

The inmate enforcers came over and asked if everything was all right.

"We're good here, guys," I reassured them.

They looked at him and said, "Hey, crazy man! You look pretty calm now. Now you see why we sent you over to Preach," one of them told him as they walked away.

Luis still had a look of amazement in his face. "Preach, so is this how God can get your attention?"

"Yes, it's definitely one of the ways. He knows your heart. He knows what troubles us. I was on the verge of killing myself, but He intervened and brought me out from that darkness and into the light. And by His Grace, I'm able to stand here with a gift He's given me to show you His work because of it."

After that, Luis asked if he could get a bunk beneath mine so I could work with him. Later that night, he told me his story. He said he'd been working in jail on his case for many years. He didn't have friends in jail or family on the outside. He was a loner. He went on for a few hours, telling me about the sadness he felt, which had begun to make him very angry around people. They just didn't really understand him, and he badly wanted them to.

After our talk, I prayed with him most of that night. After he told me his story. It seemed to calm him some. I excused myself and told him I was going over to the soda machines to buy one. His eyes lit up in amazement.

"Preach, I haven't had a sip of a soda in five years. Nobody in jail likes me. I told you I was a troublemaker, so I haven't been offered one."

The saddest look came over him, and in that moment, once again, I was seeing the little child inside all of us. Feeling hurt and pretending to be tough was him only trying to protect it.

"Luis, I've got an idea. Follow me, my brother."

I walked him over to the soda machine and asked him what was his favorite.

"Sprite! I love Sprite!" he said.

We listened to the sound of it coming down the chute, and when the plastic door opened, he just stood there. I'm not sure he knew if it was for him or not. I could tell he couldn't get past that sound I'm sure he'd heard a thousand times before and had envisioned himself drinking one. I took it from the tray and handed it to him. He just stood there and stared at it. He didn't even open it; he just continued to look at it.

"It's gonna get warm if you don't open it," I laughingly told him.

He finally did, and when he took his first sip, his face lit up like a kid watching the lights on a Christmas tree. I then bought him a bag of potato chips and he almost wouldn't take them. He said he wasn't used to anyone giving him anything.

I walked him back to the bunks and told him, "It isn't always the size of the messages God sends us—like in this case: Loren's braided cross story, a soda, or a bag of chips. It isn't the size of those gestures. It's recognizing the great source from which they come. A mustard seed of faith doesn't grow into a big tree overnight. It takes baby steps to build a relationship with God. We fall and He helps us get back up. After a while, we learn to trust Him and we find ourselves walking upright in faith—strong faith. But it has to start somewhere. And, Luis, let this moment be your first baby step. Let Him show you how to walk in that faith, as He's done for me so many times."

Over those next few weeks Luis and I became good friends. He kept his bunk below me. There was his occasional outbreak of anger toward other inmates, but they saw him changing. He'd always check himself later when he came back to his bunk. I was later transferred to another dorm. I heard he'd gotten fifty years.

THE BLOOD OF CHRIST

Troy was the inmate barber of my jail dorm. It had a population of around one hundred and thirty inmates. I didn't know what he was in for, but I realized he must have been wasting a great talent being incarcerated. He was amazing at what he did. Since the day he'd showed up a few weeks ago, the lines were long as inmates waited for him to work his magic on their heads. This was in exchange for a couple packs of peanut butter and Top Ramen, which was more valuable than money in there. He made them feel they were still on the outside, maybe preparing to go out on a date. He was able to bring their fantasies to life, maybe allowed some of them to forget for a minute they might be facing long prison terms.

Troy was a showman when he cut. I think for us it was a form of entertainment to take our minds off the drudgery of jail life and its ever-present dangers. When he finished a new head, the transformation was usually pretty miraculous. The inmate would walk over to the mirror and stare at himself as if he were Denzel preparing for his closeup.

At the end of the night, Troy would usually pick up all the hair around his area, clean the cheap, disposable razors, and collect from everyone who owed him. On this particular night, his tally was pretty hefty. He walked past me with a smile on his face as he headed toward his bunk to count the peanut butter and Top Ramen packs. I would always save my peanut butter packs from lunch. I didn't usually eat them because they tasted like cardboard and gave me serious constipation. I knew he liked them, so I stopped him and gave him the ten packs I had saved.

"Wow! What do I owe you for this?"

I told him I was giving them to him for free. I didn't charge inmates for anything.

"Thanks; I really appreciate that. My name is Troy."

"They call me, Preach," I told him.

He laughed and pointed to both of our heads.

"Yeah, with the baldheads, we look like twins," I joked.

"I've watched you preach to most of the inmates here. I've seen you break up fights with the gangs. You pass out food to inmates of all colors, and gangs who don't get commissary. That's really cool. I got a lot of respect for that, preacher man."

I thanked Troy. He then told me what he was in for and how many years he was facing. He said he was an epileptic. It made him nervous that one day somebody might not notice him having a seizure. Because he was only a few bunks away from me, I assured him I'd keep an eye on him. It made him feel better. I invited him to come to my Bible study and prayer group. He said he was "sorta into God" but hadn't been to church in years.

We were interrupted by Reggie, an inmate who was facing twenty years to life for murder, asking if I would come to his bunk and pray with him. We then left Troy to finish what he was doing.

Later that night when I'd finished praying with Reggie, I meditated for three-and-a-half hours. I needed to feel the presence of God before I prepared for prayer with a group of inmates. I talked to him about my spirit getting weary. I wasn't sure how long I'd be incarcerated.

I asked, "How long do you want me here ministering to the inmates? If it's a long time, please continue to feed my spirit with Your words, and that I may continue to spread this beautiful message and gift You have given and shown me. Amen."

The inmates were starting to come for prayer. This jail dorm was filled with quite a few gang members who had been stabbed, shot, maimed, were epileptics, you name it. Some had killed and were facing long sentences. Those same men were at the table for prayer, and some of them looked as if they'd been through quite a lot on the battlefield of street gang life. At times, during some of the group sessions, a few inmates wanted to stand up and describe how they'd gotten shot, stabbed, or maimed. Reynaldo, a Latino, stood first and took off his shirt to show where a rival gang member had taken a serrated knife and cut him from one side of his navel all the way around to the other side.

"He tried to cut me in half!" he said.

I took his hand and we all prayed for him.

Then Freddie, an African American, stood up, took off his shirt, and turned around to show us his back. After a drug deal had gone bad Freddie was chased and shot in the back, point-blank, nine times with an AK-47. He was so blessed to have lived I told him. We then prayed for him.

Next Ji-ho, a Korean, stood up. The entire left side of his head had been bashed in by a sledgehammer. He had constant tremors. He was very lucky to be alive as well. We stood and prayed for him. I wanted the guys to really understand they were still alive because of God. There was no greater relationship they could have than with the spirit of God who had saved their lives simply because He loved them. Wasn't that enough to change the path they were on? They all agreed, and some vowed to stop gang-banging if they ever got out.

As I came to the end and had all the inmates stand for the final prayer of the evening, I noticed Troy standing in the back. He'd been there for a while. He came up to me afterward and asked if I'd come to his bunk and pray with him. He walked me over and I handed him a Bible. He said he didn't have one. I showed him a few Scriptures to read later, then I prayed with him. He said the inmates' stories had really touched him. I told him the gift he had for cutting hair was bringing a lot of joy to some of the very ones at the table tonight.

In those next few weeks, Troy and I became very close. We laughed together a lot. Most of the time I'd pull up a chair and watch him work his magic on the inmates. At the end of the night, when he'd head back to his bunk exhausted, I'd always put packs of peanut butter under his pillow. He'd look over at me and, with his big infectious laugh, put his hands together as if he were praying.

I'd just finished for the night with the inmates and was doing my nightly meditations. Tonight, I wanted to let God know how grateful I was. It had been five months and my auto-immune disorder had not returned—not once! Ever since the night of the miracle. The depression was much better, especially with all the work I was doing. It kept my mind and spirit fed with His love; I had a real purpose for life now. I just couldn't stop praising Him for it. I prayed for the continued blessings for the inmates at the table and for their families' continued support for them. I could only imagine how difficult it must have been for them. I'd spoken to a few on the phone before and made a promise to them that I'd try to keep them coming to the prayer groups. I cried myself to sleep after that.

I was awakened by the ever-impressive sound of inmates of different races doing early morning gang chants and revelries. This would usually go on until every race group had gone through theirs. Things usually stayed mutually respectful, and if for some reason it didn't, whoever had been disrespectful would be seriously disciplined by men of his own race. That would usually involve at least ten or more inmates stomping him out in a corner.

The jail dorm was now bustling. Card games at the foot of inmate's bunks. The sound of baseball blaring on the TV. Inmates begging for coffee. Brawls. The norm. I went in to use the restroom, which was a large, open room with a long urinal for everyone. There was a mirror right in the front of it which was used for shaving. As I stood there, I suddenly saw a vision flash in front of me. It was Troy falling off his top bunk. Within that next minute, there was a loud thud, followed by inmates yelling!

"Oh my God!"

"He just fell!"

I just knew it was Troy. God had just warned me. When I ran into the room I had to work my way through all the inmates who were scattering away from the scene. Troy was lying there in a large pool of blood and not moving.

"God, please let him be alive," I prayed. I couldn't understand why no-one in the room was trying to help him. Then it hit me: they were afraid they might contract AIDS. The pool of blood was starting to get larger. I ran over to Troy and dropped on my knees into it. Blood splashed all over my arm. Some of it was now spreading and going under some of the bunks. The inmates were still jumping out of the way of it. He wasn't moving and I couldn't feel a pulse. *'Is he dead?'* I wasn't a doctor, so I wasn't sure. I didn't want to move him either, because if his neck was broken it might cause more damage.

His best friend Sonny was standing behind me, yelling at the top of his lungs.

"Preach! You can't let him die! He's my best friend!"

Sonny said he had been trying to get off his bunk and had had an epileptic seizure mid-air. That was when he'd hit the ground, head first. And with him being bald, I noticed a split where he hit his head. This was where the blood was oozing from. I felt his pulse again—still nothing.

I yelled out, "Does anyone in here know CPR?"

There was no response. Nobody wanted to chance it. I knew from being in there that it could take up to a half-an-hour for the paramedics to arrive. They weren't on the jail premises; they had to be dispatched. Sonny kept yelling for me not to let him die, so I did what God had brought me there to do: pray.

"Dear Father God, as I sit here on my knees in a pool of blood of such a gifted young man, there's a chance he might be dead. I'm not a doctor, but I am a prayer warrior, and this blood isn't tainted from AIDS. I'm not claiming that fear! I'm claiming it as 'the Blood of Christ'. Please, God, touch him and don't let him die. Please bring another miracle for these inmates to witness."

I opened my eyes from the prayer and smacked Troy in his face as hard as I could. Suddenly, his hand twitched. I repeated it again and his body started to slowly move, but his eyes were still closed. I didn't know if he had been dead in those last few minutes or just been knocked out. Only God knew that answer. But then he started moving.

"Preach!" Sonny yelled out. "He moved! Thank God, he's moving!"

By this time, the guards and paramedics had come rushing in and were ordering everyone to their bunks. "Immediately!" they shouted. We ran to our bunks and watched as the paramedics and guards surrounded Troy. A few minutes later, he was whisked away. I went into prayer for him, and the dorm soon went back to normal. I just sat there and kept praying.

"Show them a miracle," I asked God. "Let Troy walk back into this dorm today. You are a God of immense love, compassion, and grace, and I claim the knowing of it from my own experiences. But there are those present who may not be Believers, Lord. Please help them to become Believers as You done for me. In the name of your loving son I pray. Amen."

Normally, when an inmate had any medical emergency, especially as tragic as Troy's, they never returned to the dorm. They were transferred and their bunk was immediately reassigned. I wasn't going to claim any of that for Troy. God told me he was coming back. The prophecy of his miracle would be fulfilled, and I held to that belief while sitting there for hours, meditating and praying for him.

There was a sudden tap on my bunk and I opened my eyes. It was Sonny, with a smile on his face, bigger than a child getting her first bike for Christmas.

"Preach! Troy's over there! He's alive!"

Sonny almost snatched me off my top bunk from his excitement. I followed him over and, sitting there with a brace on his neck, was Troy.

"It was Preach who prayed for you, Troy," he told him.

He reached his hand out to thank me.

"I'm only the messenger, my brother," I reminded him as I pointed my finger up to God.

He looked puzzled as he started telling everyone around him that it was very strange. He had gone somewhere while he was lying in his blood.

I told him. "It wasn't your blood anymore in that moment. It was 'the Blood of Christ' you were in. That's who saved you, my friend."

I reached behind my back, handed him a few packs of peanut butter, and left him with his friends. He had a big grin on his face. Only God knew what really had happened to Troy during the time he was unresponsive. It remains a mystery to this day.

It couldn't have been more than an hour later and Troy was back at his cutting station with the neck brace still on and a big patch on the side of his head. It wasn't going to stop him from doing what he did best, and that was making the inmates' lives just a little bit better.

DECEMBER 19TH

I talked to my sister that day and she put my mother on three-way. She was in good spirits, as usual. I thanked them for the support of my jail ministry. My family had put money on my books every other week since I'd been incarcerated. It had allowed me to feed the ones that didn't have family on the outside, or the ones who'd forgotten them. They were always grateful. It was important to show them God's symbolic love for them.

We had just finished lunch in the jail dorm, and the trustees were taking away the last of the trays when Dre, the dorm leader, yelled out from across the room to me.

"Preach! Got another one I'm sending over."

That's when a young black inmate limped over to my bunk. He looked beaten up pretty badly. "Wow! What happened to you?" I asked.

He introduced himself as James. Then he asked why he had been sent over to me. I told him, in the condition he was in, he looked like he was in bad need of prayer.

"Nice to meet you. Preach, right? I was sent over from another dorm. It was filled with a lot of gang members. Some of them tried to gang rape me. When I resisted, I got jumped. That's when my mother found out and they threatened my life! So, they sent me to another dorm. It looks like there're gang members in this one as well."

"Most jails have gang members, but I try to break up most of the fights here. Somehow, they trust me. I'm sure they won't try to rape you in an open dorm like this. James, do you really believe you're here by accident? Did Dre tell you what I do here? I preach and give the Word to inmates. Some are distressed more than others, like yourself. This is when I know God has sent them directly to me."

"Really? Wow! That's great."

"I know you probably don't believe that, right? So, God's telling me right now He's going to give you a sign. He's telling me you used to do prayer for the inmates in the dorms you were in. That you want to learn how to meditate and need someone to help teach you how to become closer to Him. The sign He's giving you right now is... me and your father have something in common."

"What's that?"

"When is your father's birthday and how old is he?"

"He's fifty-nine and was born on December 19, 1953."

"That's the exact same day and year I was born. We're the same age."

"No way! That's just not possible. You have to prove that to me."

"James, there're three hundred sixty-five days in a year, and your dad's could have been on any one of those, right? He could've been any age, right?

There're nineteen thousand inmates here. So, think about it: what are the odds of any of those things happening?"

I took him to my bunk, and sorted through my papers until I found a court document, proving it to him. I knew God had James's attention at this point. This poor young man was in jail for something he said he'd done that was stupid. He said he'd known better and was probably facing a few years for it.

"Preach, now that God has my attention, what does He have planned for me?"

"Well, that's between you and God on that question. Maybe when you learn to meditate—clearing the mind from chatter—and become closer in the Word, maybe it will help you to find that true purpose. Especially if you feel this might be it. I know there's definitely one for you because of some of the trials you're facing now. In the book of James 1:1-5, it reads: *My brethren, count it all joy when you fall into various trials, knowing that the testing of your faith produces patience. But let patience have its perfect work, that you may be perfect and complete, lacking nothing.*"

James was starting to see part of the work it was going to take on his journey. He was a quick learner. We spent hours every day deep in meditation and learning the Word together. He was enjoying freely ministering to the inmates in the dorm, where he didn't have to worry about being gang raped or beat down.

I remember the day he called to tell his mother. She was crying joyous tears for him. She said, at first with him being in jail, she had been frightened for his life, especially after the incident, but now he was praying with inmates, meditating, and doing what she knew he'd always wanted to do on the outside. Now he was doing God's work in a place where it was so much more greatly needed. He had a purpose. I could tell by the look on his face after he hung up with her that she was so proud of him.

Most of the time, when inmates accepted a plea deal, they weren't in the dorm much longer after that, so when James got back from court, I knew his time was limited in the dorm. He'd been sentenced to two years. In those next few days, we ended the last of our praying and meditating, and I knew in my heart he was ready to take on God's work. His relationship was building so beautifully and I could feel the confidence from his spirit.

"James, I'm gonna miss you, my friend. We got the chance to do a lot of great work together. I just know God's going to do some amazing things with you."

"Yeah, Preach, it was great. Thanks so much. You really freaked me out about you and my dad being born on the same day and year." We had a good laugh. "All I can say is, I'm learning that God works in mysterious ways."

James turned and waved as he walked out the door. He was carrying his duffel bag, but the most important thing he carried was God's Word in his spirit. I knew He'd sent me one after another to bring them closer to Him, and I had been so grateful to help him receive the sign that I myself had received.

It's Called Hope

I was having a late Bible study that day, when this young Latino inmate sat down at the Spyder table with us. The aura of his spirit felt lost and his face seemed a bit swollen. I wasn't sure if he'd been beaten up or had done it to himself. Some of the inmates had just come off suicide watch, and there were often visible indications of physical violence they had inflicted on themselves. I'd never seen him in the dorm before, but God was telling me he needed prayer badly. He didn't know it yet, but that was why he was there. Throughout the study, he seemed fascinated by the words. After it was over, he stayed around and began asking questions.

"Hi, sir; my name is Jordan Jimenez."

"Nice to meet you, Jordan. My name is Robert Palmer, but here they call me Preach. Do you believe in God?"

"I'm not sure. I was standing next to the table and overheard what you were preaching about. It got my attention and that's why I came over."

"Well, God's glad you're here, my young brother. How old are you?"

"I recently turned nineteen. They just released me off suicide watch a couple of days ago."

"Do you still plan to kill yourself?"

"I'm not sure. I'm still really depressed."

He said they'd put him on meds, but he wasn't sure if they were working yet. I sensed there was something much deeper bothering Jordan. That's when he broke down and started crying, and told me, "I spoke to my mom a few days ago, and she gave me the worse news I've ever got in my young life. She told me my girlfriend Amanda had a miscarriage! She was only two months pregnant!"

"Oh my God!" I said. That's when he just let it all go.

"What do I do, Preach? I'm not gonna make it through this. My first child is now dead! That was the best thing that's ever happened to my life. Poor Amanda. I can't imagine what she's going through right now. I've been addicted to heroin for a while now and I thought this was going to help me quit. I just wish I wasn't here. If I was on the outside I could go out and get high, and try to kill myself again!"

I took him to my cell and prayed for Jordan. I knew that was the only way he was going to make it through the night. He looked at me with swollen eyes and broken spirit and said, "Preach, what makes you think God can help me get through this?"

"Jordan, it's called hope. It's called compassion. It's called grace. God knows our pain. I went through life always feeling like I was in control, until something tragic happened that took it away. I didn't know who else to lean on at that moment. That's when the voice of God said, 'I will never forsake you.' What that means is, God will never give up on us no matter what we're going through. Like you right now. It only takes a mustard seed of faith in Him, and from there, the miracles begin to happen.

"Trust me, my young brother, I am a living and breathing witness to that love and strength He can provide. When we release and let go of our pain, we give it to Him. That's when He can touch places deep inside us that no one else can reach, to heal our wounds."

I told Jordan that was what I was praying for him.

"Why don't you let me help you start a relationship with Him? You see, I learned to rely on Him to help get me through those challenging days, like the ones you're facing now. See, here, look at my wrists. I'm here preaching to inmates like yourself, because when I meditate and read His Word, it keeps my mind and spirit out of the darkness and suicidal thoughts. His Word is very healing. I tell you it really works. Do you have a Bible?"

"No, I don't."

"Here, take this one. Let me read you some Scriptures I believe are a good place for us to start."

In those next few days, Jordan told me about his family and how he'd worked at a bakery with his mom. She'd always wanted him to have a relationship with God, but he really didn't want to listen to her. He would just resort to doing heroin again.

"I've really been fighting hard to kick this heroin habit. Do you think God can help me with it?"

I told him there were plenty of programs he could join when he got out, but while he was in jail, yes, God could help him start.

"Jordan, when you stick a needle in your arm to shoot heroin, don't you wait and trust it will eventually get you high?"

He nodded yes.

"So, I'm asking you to inject God's love into your spirit in place of it. Give Him that same trust you give to heroin for it to work. If you're willing to replace the high from heroin with God, I promise the only side effects you'll have are love, grace, redemption, and His undying compassion for you. Not the insidious gratification from heroin."

I asked Jordan to let me teach him how to let God show how much He loved him, in the same way He'd shown me when I was a hard drug addict and had overdosed. I told him how I'd had a hard attack and died back in 1985, but had been clean ever since. It was an amazing God I'd discovered at that time. He had brought me back to life. I'd tried trusting him instead of drugs. I was now myself beginning to understand one of His reasons why. He had a purpose for me in this life. Maybe to stand there at that moment with Jordan, telling that story, so that he could learn to trust God's love for himself.

After that day, he showed up at my bunk at five every morning to learn the Word of God. I even showed him how to meditate. He said his need for not wanting heroin was getting better. God was taking its place. I told him he still needed to join a program along with building his relationship with God, for extra support. We did a lot of praying together, and I could now feel the aura of his spirit brightening and pushing up through the darkness that had been present on the first day I'd met Jordan. He said his suicidal thoughts were starting to leave and he was happy because he was going to court that next day. It looked like he might be getting out soon. He was really hoping to.

But everything came crashing down on Jordan that next evening when he returned from court. He said he'd found out Amanda had run away from his parents' home. She was very distraught over the miscarriage. She was nowhere to be found, and they were very worried about her. It was time for lights out in the jail dorm and the inmates were preparing for sleep. I could tell Jordan was going to have a rough night on his own. His spirit was crushed. I had him come to my cell. As we sat there on the cold floor throughout the night, I reminded him of all the work we'd done over those past few weeks.

"Jordan, now is the time for you to see how important it is to trust God in these kinds of moments I told you about. When we have no control over our situations, He's all we have to depend on. All He needs from you right now is that mustard seed of faith you've started growing inside you these past few weeks. Let Him take care of the rest."

Jordan finally fell asleep. Somehow it seemed comforting enough to get him through one more night of grief. Me, I kept praying for him.

"God, I have no idea what this child of yours is going through right now. What I do know is, his spirit needs healing from the love that only You can provide him. Please come to him and let him feel Your presence in his moment of loneliness and despair. Assuage his pain. Give his family the comfort they're praying for. Wherever his girlfriend is, please touch her spirit and provide her with protection in the streets. Give her the strength she needs for the loss of their child. Please return her safely to his parents' home. There isn't a person on this earth You feel isn't just as special as him. I know You are no respecter of persons, but I pray in this moment for You to give him favor, so that his spirit feels he is truly special. Father, he needs You tonight. Amen."

That next morning, Jordan said he felt he had been touched again by God's spirit. "Preach, it felt comforting. I'm beginning to feel God really does love me. I can feel that mustard seed of faith you planted with me starting to grow."

"Yes, he does, my brother, and it only gets better. Our heart can only love as much as we allow it. Let us learn a godly love, which is abundant and bountiful."

Jordan went to court that next day. I noticed he had left a letter on my bunk. It was him thanking me for the beautiful experience he'd had learning about God. My heart was full at that moment. He'd left his info as well. Jordan was released from court and never came back that day. That was the last time I ever saw him.

Years later, one day on Father's Day, I was sitting in my studio when a message popped up on Facebook Messenger. It was Jordan, thanking me for bringing him to God, saying he'd been off heroin the entire time and his life was in a great place. He was still reading his Bible and praying. I told him how proud I was of him and that he should continue to keep Him in his life. It had all started for him with a tiny mustard seed of faith. Now see how much it had grown.

Below is his letter. I typed it out from the handwritten one, but left it in his exact words:

FROM MISERY TO HOPE

WHEN I FIRST CAME INTO TWIN TOWER COUNTY JAIL, I WAS A MESS.
I WAS PUT ON THE 7TH LEVEL OF TOWER TWO, WHICH IS SUICIDE WATCH.
I HAD A PREGNANT GIRLFRIEND 2 MONTHS INTO HER PREGNANCY, AND A MOTHER WHO IS VERY
DEPRESSED. SO NEEDLESS TO SAY I HAD A LOT ON MY MIND AND THIS GAVE ME MANY WORRIES IN MY
HEAD, AND DROVE ME CRAZY. SO I ENDED UP BEATING MYSELF UP LITERALLY GAVE MYSELF SWOLLEN
FACE, BLACK-EYE.

ON MY 3RD DAY ON THE SEVENTH FLOOR I ASKED GOD FOR A WAY TO CALM MYSELF THROUGH ALL
MY WORRIES.

NEXT DAY I WAS MOVED TO THE 6TH FLOOR A-POD. STILL FELT DOWN WORRIED MANY NEGATIVE
THOUGHTS, MANY SUICIDAL. THAT NIGHT I WAS MOVED TO A-POD.
I WAS WOKEN AROUND 2:00 AM AND MOVED TO C-POD. BEING DEPRESSED AND ALL I WAS TRYING TO
BE STRONG FOR MY FAMILY, AND MY PREGNANT GIRLFRIEND. NOW IT WORKED FOR TWO DAYS.

THEN I GOT ONE OF THE WORSE NEWS ANYBODY CAN HEAR IN JAIL. MY GIRLFRIEND HAD A
MISCARRIAGE, AND THIS DROVE ME IN A DEEP DEPRESSION. AND THIS VERY WISEMAN TOOK NOTICE
AND HIS NAME WAS ROBERT PALMER, AND ONE NIGHT AFTER DINNER HE WAS HAVING HIS BIBLE
STUDY WITH THE INMATES. IT CAUGHT MY ATTENTION. I SAT DOWN TO LISTEN TO HIS WORDS. THEY
SPOKE TO ME AND WORKED WONDERS AND LET ME SLEEP THAT NIGHT.

NEXT FEW DAYS I GOT NEWS THAT MY GIRLFRIEND RAN AWAY FROM HOME. OH MAN WORDS COULD
NOT DESCRIBE HOW BAD I FELT, NOR HOW MANY TEARS I SHED. I FELT HOPELESS,LOST,DEPRESSED.
MAN, NO ONES WORDS COULD COMFORT ME NOT EVEN MY OWN MOTHER'S.

SO FINALLY I HAD ASKED ROBERT TO LISTEN TO MY PROBLEMS, HE DID AND JUST BY HIS KINDNESS
TO LISTEN TO MY PROBLEMS OVER HIS OWN, CAUGHT ME AND EVEN SHOCKED ME. SO I CAME TO HIM
OVER A COUPLE OF WEEKS. HE PRAYED WITH ME FOR MY MOTHER AND GIRLFRIEND. HE LISTENED TO
WHAT I HAD TO SAY. GOT ME A BIBLE, SLOWLY MADE ME BELIEVE AND GROW HOPE, AND BUILD A
RELATIONSHIP WITH GOD

AND IT'S BEEN HELPING ME PASS THROUGH THESE SAD AND WORRYING TIMES, EVEN THOUGH I
STILL HAVEN'T HEARD FROM MY GIRLFRIEND, WHO I LOVE AND CARE FOR EXTREMELY. I GROWN
CLOSER TO MY MOTHER AND FATHER. GOT A PLAN TO CHANGE MY HEROIN DRUG HABITS SINCE I GOT
MORE AND MORE OF A REASON TO FIGHT EVERYDAY, WITH THREE WEEKS TO GO UNTIL MY NEXT
COURT DATE, AND HOPEFULLY RELEASE DAY.

I THANK THE WISEST MAN I EVER MET, ROBERT PALMER FOR HIS TIME AND AMAZING WORDS
BRINGING ME CLOSER TO GOD.

THE GARDEN

I had now been incarcerated for about ten months, ministering to maybe over nine hundred inmates in quite a few dorms in the L.A. County Jail. This had become my home for now. I had no idea when I was leaving and somehow didn't care. I was still on God's mission. Even after doing it for seven days a week that entire time, I still felt His work hadn't been completed yet. There were still more souls that needed saving, and as long as He was gracious enough to continue to give me this gift and the breath each morning to use it, I was willing to start over again tomorrow.

This was that tomorrow, and I'd woken up breathing again. The day was just getting started and we'd just finished breakfast—a small box of cereal, a half-pint of milk, and a banana. That would be it until lunch, and if you were used to eating a lot on the outside, in here you'd definitely shed the weight you'd fought your entire life to lose.

There seemed to be more of a traffic flow of new fish (inmates) than usual coming up for prayer. I always welcomed it and I'm sure God did too. So, I went longer than normal, and afterward tried to get at least a few hours of meditation in before it got busy again. It was during that meditation that an inmate tapped my bunk. I opened my eyes and he was staring at me with a look on his face like he wanted to kill me. His energy was very dark and I knew because of the jail dorm I was in, he could easily be facing a murder charge. If so, I would minister to him anyway. I'd gotten used to it by then. It didn't bother me anymore. That was why God had me there. Little did he know that maybe this was the meeting he needed to make with Him today.

"Why did they send me over to you?" he hollered at me.

"I'm not sure. Who sent you over?" I asked calmly.

He turned and pointed across the room to the dorm leader Ren, who pointed back at him, confirming having sent him over.

It was something the dorm leaders had gotten used to doing with me. It was when a strange bird, as they called them, came in with a disruptive attitude. If I couldn't spiritually calm them down, they'd sometimes send a squad over to stomp them out, then drop them at the front door. I'd always try to help avoid that option. I knew they still had their eyes on this one. I gave them the usual sign that I was good and to give me a chance with him. They nodded back.

"What's your name?" I asked him.

"My name's Herman."

"They call me, Preach."

"So, Preach, tell me what it is you do, so I can tell you if you can even help me."

I asked him if he believed in God. He said, "It depends." I asked him what was bothering him. He said he wanted to keep it short.

"You're the last person I will talk to about this, because that inmate over there who sent me here said you could talk me out of doing something crazy."

I asked what it was.

"When I leave here tomorrow I'm going straight to my girlfriend's house. Then I'm going to kill her."

"It's not my business, Herman, why you would want to do that, but if I can pray with you, at least while you're here to try to help change your mind, please let me try. I really think when you get out of here you need to check yourself in somewhere for professional help before you do something you might be sorry for."

Herman just looked at me, then asked for me to pray for him. I asked him to close his eyes and give me his hands. I knew he was nervous because he kept looking around the room and couldn't focus. His hands were very rough and still shaking.

"Let me help you calm your spirit first, Herman?" I asked him.

He quickly yanked his hands away from me. Gently, I took them back and had him close his eyes again. He soon calmed down and relaxed himself.

"Murder is a strong word, my friend. I can't imagine what happened to make you feel you'd want to commit something so dark, and it's not my business."

"Because she deserves it!"

I knew I was running out of time with Herman, and he was running out of patience with me. His eyes were still closed and the shaking had started again. I prayed for him for a few minutes. He opened his eyes and said he still hadn't changed his mind.

"Stay with me here," I told him. I asked him to close his eyes again for me. I then prayed to God for help with this lost one. His spirit just seemed hell-bent on murder, despite me sharing with him in as many ways as possible that murder was a sin. He still didn't care. I took his hands with mine and started moving them in an up-and-down, digging motion.

"What are we doing?" he asked, confused.

"Just stay with me, my brother. Herman, your spirit's broken, like mine was. When I lost my way, God was the only One in this world who could help me. Do you think I've always been here, preaching to lost souls? No, I was one myself. I'm still working on getting better myself. It's a lifetime process, but with God in our lives, it makes it a lot easier to understand the things we don't. Just look at my wrists if you don't believe that God really understands our pain. It was He who brought me out of the darkness when I tried to kill myself. In a way, I was taking a life He created. It's no different than what you're talking about doing to your girlfriend. We don't have the right to kill one of His creations, neither one of us. We both should respect that precious work He's done, right?"

I kept trying to convince Herman. I told him I didn't know what he was personally going through, to want to kill someone, but God knew what had happened to make him this angry. His spirit had hardened and the inner child felt unprotected. I had done the same thing to my own.

"Herman, God knows that's who's truly suffering, so try not to blame yourself. You're just the man who wants to protect him at any cost but hasn't quite learned how to yet, without taking it out in a hurtful way on someone else. And now maybe killing them. That kind of anger stops when you stop hurting him first, your inner-child."

Both of our eyes were still closed, but I could feel the cloud over Herman's dark spirit beginning to lift. I held his hands even tighter and assured him I wasn't going to let him go. "Don't worry, God's got you, my brother. He's got both of us. He doesn't want either one of us killing anybody, especially that little boy inside us who's suffered the most."

That's when I took both of our hands and started a digging motion, as if I were planting something. I repeated the digging motion, then I said, "Herman, what we're doing is letting God dig a deep hole in the ground of that anger inside you. He wants to reach that inner child and plant seeds of love in his heart, as He's done for mine before. The tears that are now streaming down my face are watering the soil, so it can begin to grow within your broken spirit. He will continue to water it with you, as long as you're willing to let Him, only this time with your own tears of love, and not the anger and rage that's burning inside you."

Herman opened his eyes. He didn't say a word. A small smile was trying to form on his face. It spoke volumes. My hopes were that God had touched him. I told him, when they released him tomorrow, to please get some professional help if he continued to have the desire to kill his girlfriend. He nodded, went over, and sat on his bunk. Then, he got into a lotus position, like I was when we'd first met. He looked over at me, almost as if to ask if he was doing it right. I nodded, and he closed his eyes and started meditating. I had hoped something had moved inside of him. I really felt for him. How could I not have? I had no idea how he'd gotten to that point in his life—only my own journey there—and in knowing that, it allowed me to show him compassion.

I was hoping he wasn't going to still kill anyone. God had hopefully released that poor inner child from the grips of his anger, as He had done for me, and Jordan was now in His hands. I knew we were still in the real world and it was going to take a lot of time—most likely years—of professional help, for him to totally let go and begin to let God in. It wasn't going to happen overnight, but this was a good place for him to start from. Just knowing that was comforting.

My work was done here. I couldn't do anymore, but I knew God could, and there were professionals out there. Hopefully, Herman didn't need to be his little inner child's abusive protector anymore. He could now let God embrace him with His unwavering love and teach him how to accept being one of His children, a man allowing forgiveness and compassion to start growing in his new garden.

A Sign For Michael

When I first met Michael Palmer in L.A. County Jail, it was in the 9400 dorms. I was in the middle of my morning meditation. When I finished, I looked over and noticed a lot of new inmates had just arrived. A couple of bunks over from me was this black inmate, reading his Bible. I got his attention and told him God had told me he and I had something in common. I could tell he was taken aback by it.

"What's your name?" I asked.

"Michael Palmer."

I told him mine was Robert Palmer. He said he didn't believe it, so I came over and showed him my wrist band. He was shocked! I also told him there would be more signs for him. I went back over to my bunk and finished meditating. When I finished this time, I looked over and told Michael it was happening again. God was giving him another sign. He was reading his Bible, but I wasn't aware of what Scripture it was. My Bible was on my bunk in front of me, facing from the back. Without looking, I stuck my index finger around the front of it on a random page. Holding the cover open from the back with my thumb, I got up, went over to Mike, and told him to look at where my finger was in the Bible. I still couldn't see where it was.

"Wow! No way! It's on Matthew 23:4, exactly the same spot I'm reading!"

I told Mike these were signs for him. God wanted his attention, so he could help me provide for the inmates some of the things to uplift their spirits, not bring it down the way this disgusting place was doing. Let them see that God does exist. They needed to know He was there for them despite it. After that, Mike had his bunk changed next to mine so we could do prayer work together. In those passing weeks, we did a lot of praying and Bible study. It helped deal with our own personal lives and we helped a lot of inmates. God's presence was definitely in the dorm, and I knew at times even Mike felt it. It wasn't long before we became good friends.

One morning, we were awakened by an intense heat that had enveloped the room. Inmates were crying out and banging on doors as they yelled to get out. The heat was now unbearable; it had to be at least 120°F in there. Epileptics were passing out at the door and some were having seizures, but nobody walked over to help them. Panicked voices were yelling, "Let us out of here! Open the doors! We can't breathe!"

The guard came over the intercom saying a transformer had blown out for the entire area on that block. The backup generators were down as well. Because we were in a high-security, twenty-four/seven locked-down dorm, there was nothing they could do until it came back on. And they didn't have an idea when that would be. We were told it was now in the low-one hundreds outside, and we knew the temperature was still steadily rising in the dorm. We were drenched in sweat.

A few epileptics started to convulse. One fell face first, hitting the concrete. That's when I grabbed Mike and had him help me keep them from swallowing their tongues. We couldn't chance letting them die or getting brain damage. The heat generated from one hundred ten inmates made it swelter even more. They finally opened one door and put a fan in front of it. But after a while it just made things worse, so, they turned it off and closed the door.

We got the epileptics taken care of. Some inmates in my Bible group agreed to watch them, but something had to be done, and quick. I had an idea. When Mike and I received weekly commissary, we fed inmates who didn't usually receive anything from their families. Sometimes there would be a piece of cardboard left in the pack. We searched through the old packs and couldn't find one. That's when Mike remembered he had a legal pad.

"Let's turn this into a few small fans and go out into the dorm and fan the inmates. Let's say a prayer and get started," I told them, knowing none of us three had a drop of energy to spare.

We went out into the dorm, started at one end, and went up and down the rows of bunks to each inmate, regardless of gang affiliation or ethnic background. We fanned him for a few minutes until he was dry, then went on to the next one. They couldn't believe it. I think they thought we were crazy at first, but they were very grateful. We repeated this for four-and-a-half hours without a break, going around the entire dorm over forty times. We kept fanning the inmates until the transformers finally came back on.

It took late into the night to finally get the temperature back down. After that, more than one hundred inmates waited to get in showers that held only four at a time. Later, some of them came over to our bunks to thank us. It was very gratifying for Mike and me. I told him it was an honor to do God's work with him.

A few days after that incident, Mike was transferred to another dorm. Things didn't seem the same around there for a few days after he'd left. I missed our work together and the pure joy it had brought me to see us both getting closer to God.

A few years passed and I called Mike. I asked him if he remembered what had happened back there in L.A. County Jail.

"How could I ever forget it!" he said.

"Just believe!"

The day Lance arrived at the dorm, it was in a very hectic state. Fights were breaking out every day. Some inmates were overdosing from crushing and snorting their meds. He came over to me and introduced himself. I told him my real name, but said they called me Preach. He immediately began to make his bed, but you could instantly tell he was pretty pissed off about something. Lance seemed like a nice guy. He was black and looked to be in his late fifties with salt-and-pepper hair.

He said he'd been on the street riding his bike when a patrol car pulled him over for no reason he could think of. He said they questioned him and told him he was under arrest. Then they cuffed him and put him in the car. He asked the officers why they were arresting him. He said they didn't respond. They just drove away with him in the back and left his bike on the street. He told them he needed to go by his house to lock his sliding glass door. They didn't care, he said. They just brought him straight to the station and booked him.

He said he'd been to jail plenty of times, but this was strange. He'd never been arrested and not given a reason, and he'd demanded his rights. The only problem for Lance was that they kept ignoring him. That's when I told him maybe this time God was trying to tell him something. He looked at me like I was crazy.

I told him, "I don't expect you to understand me, not just yet, but in time it will be revealed to you. Lance, sometimes when we feel we're in control, God has to show us we aren't, so we can learn how to depend on Him for our needs. It also is a way to build a relationship with Him."

Lance ignored me. I didn't expect him to understand—I didn't at first—but I was determined to show him a sign from God to change his mind.

"Lance, do you believe in God?"

"Yes, I do, Preach."

"Do you have faith? If your faith is truly strong, you can leave here anytime you want."

After hearing that and just having met me, he really thought I was crazy. I laughed.

"Preach, no disrespect, but what does that have to do with me? And, if you believe that, then why are you still here?"

"That's a great question, Lance. Maybe it's simply to stand here in this minute to tell you what I just did, and in time, show you how real He is. If that's God's only purpose for me being in here, to me it's a purpose well served."

After that, he had me talk to him about faith. I did for about an hour, but I could still see his skepticism.

Days passed and Lance still hadn't been released. By this point he was so frustrated and I knew he was at his limit. He paced the floor, wondering when they were going to release him. I wanted to share with Lance, in hopes it would change the way he looked at faith, but I could tell he was losing ground on that subject. I felt God was soon going to reveal Himself to him.

That time came a few days later at about two in the morning. I'd just returned to my bunk from praying with an inmate who was very distraught over his wife leaving him. Most of the inmates in the dorm were asleep and the lights were dim. Lance was pacing the floors between our bunks. He'd been there for a while now, and things still hadn't changed for him. He still didn't know when he was leaving. I knew God was trying to reach him, but he wasn't listening. That's when I looked at him and called him over to my bunk.

He walked up, frustrated, and said, "I just don't get it. I've been here all this time. Why isn't anybody telling me anything?"

"Lance, I know you don't believe me when I tell you God wants you to listen to Him. You're here because you don't have faith. He wants to help you restore it. Please trust me when I tell you this."

"Preach, I just can't see how that's connected to me. I told you that just sounds too crazy for me to believe. I mean, come on. If I told that to somebody in here or on the outside, they'd think I was crazy!"

That's when I knew God was telling me He was going to give him a sign. Right at that moment, Jose, a Latino inmate, ran over and sat at the foot of Lance's bunk to witness what he'd seen before in the dorm.

"Lance, do you want to leave? I'm going to show you the kind of faith you have to have. Watch this."

I cupped my hand to my ear, and at that very second, over the loudspeaker came the command, "Lance Johnson, roll it up for release!"

Lance yelled out, "No way, Preach! That is impossible! That is physically impossible! How'd you do that?"

He grabbed me with tears streaming down his eyes, still in disbelief. Jose grabbed me and started praying. He also was deeply moved by it.

"It's simply called faith," I kept telling him. "Trusting God that everything is working in your favor. Now do you understand what I was preaching to you, about how I'd lost mine? There were signs along the way that helped me restore it. I just needed to go deeper into faith and meditation to build my faith, and to listen."

He started talking fast and saying, "I can't wait to get on back on the street to tell my family and friends what I witnessed watching you pray with the inmates about faith. I just know they're not going to believe me."

"You know what, Lance, maybe it isn't for them to believe. Maybe it was God talking directly to you. You're the one here who needs to believe it. I believe He deals with each of us differently."

While he packed his bags to leave, he kept saying, "I'm just stunned! Stunned!"

He kept shaking his head and repeating it as the door unlocked to let him out. He turned and said, "Preach, here, take my name and information, just in case somebody doesn't believe this really happened."

As the door closed behind him, something was telling me that Lance was going to go back to believing again, maybe even more so now after what he'd just witnessed. *'I couldn't have made that up,'* I thought. I knew it in my heart. I headed back to my bunk. Jose was still there. He'd seen how God had worked before and was smiling as he said goodnight and returned to his own bed.

THE JAR FILLED WITH HAPPINESS

The day Ray arrived at the jail dorm, he was walking around looking for a bunk. The ones in ours were extremely rusted and mildewed, and they had to be wired together just to keep from breaking down. They were so close that if you turned sideways, you'd hit another inmate and hopefully not one with a horrible staph infection all over his body. If you were unfortunate to be on a bottom bunk, all you saw was one long continuous dark dungeon of bunks and the arms of sleeping inmates dangling like corpses in a morgue.

I told Ray he was fortunate because the bunk next to me was open. God was bringing me another one for a lesson. I could see he was carrying quite a few duffel bags.

"Do you need help with any of those?" I asked him.

"No, I'm good; thanks. My name is Ray," he held out his hand and said. "I've been sentenced already and I'm just waiting to get transferred to prison. Unfortunately, they never tell you when that day will be. It can be weeks or months. You just hear your name called over the loudspeaker one day and you'd better be at the front door in ten minutes. I can't wait to get out of this hellhole. I've never liked coming to this place; they'll kill you in here. You gotta always watch ya back. Prisons are more chilled; plus, you get hot meals."

"They call me Preach," I told him.

Ray jumped up on his bunk and started sorting through his bags. Within minutes, his entire bunk was scattered with spiritual pamphlets, hair products, a Bible... he'd come at the right time because we were just getting ready for chow.

"What do you guys get served on Friday?" he asked.

"You're in luck. Breaded chicken patties. This is the only day out of the week the food is halfway decent," I jokingly told him.

On any other day, it was usually something mysterious that they called 'meat', floating in soggy noodles of grease. The food trustees were starting to make their rounds. At this time, all the inmates had to lay on their stomachs at the foot of the bunk to get their trays. When the trustee walked by with the cart filled with milk cartons, he accidentally forgot to give Ray one.

"Hey, punk! You forgot me!" he yelled out.

"Here you can have mine," I whispered to him.

(I knew you weren't supposed to talk directly to the trustees. It could get the entire food program shut down for the night. The sheriffs frequently made that very clear.)

"Hey! You forgot me!" he yelled out again. "Don't make me have to come down there and grab one from you!"

At this point, the trustee didn't quite know how to respond, so I gave Ray mine. He kept insisting the trustee give him the one owed to him. After a few minutes, he finally backed down and took mine. He later told me he was tired of having people in jail trying to take advantage of him. I told him I didn't think that was what the trustee was trying to do, but Ray insisted, so we let it go for the night. He said he knew he had a temper.

"It gets the best of me sometimes," he said. "I'm just not going to let anybody do that."

Once again, I felt God had put Ray there for a reason that was unknown to both of us at that point.

I had my prayer group after chow. The inmates all came around my bunk with their Bibles. I asked Ray if he wanted to join.

"No, I think I'm gonna just read."

As he was reading his Bible, he seemed slightly irritated by all the inmates around my bunk. I could tell that all the voices around him were getting to be too much. He jumped down and went to watch TV. Within minutes, he got into it with another inmate. When he came back, I asked him to share with me what he'd gotten from reading his Bible.

He said, "Comfort."

I felt I could not argue with someone's interpretation of the Word, but I was willing to challenge him on how he applied it. He said he'd been in and out of jail his entire life, and it was all he knew—fighting and defending himself.

"Do you ever give it a chance to work?" I asked.

"What do you mean by that?"

"By you giving first and not expecting anything in return. Even in this wretched place, it can be done. It's a state of mind and consciousness," I shared with him. "That's where we can apply what we're reading."

"But then people will start to use you in here. I saw you give those inmates some of your commissary. Why? That just makes them keep coming back for more. Watch; you'll see. I've been coming here too long, my brother."

"Ray, I can't be used. You wanna know why? Because I give it to God first, and it's Him who gives it to them. When I share the food with the inmates, it somehow brings them to Him and not the food. To them, it creates a more symbolic feeling of His love for them. For me, that is so much more gratifying than wondering if I'm being used every time they come over and ask me for anything. So, I'm able to freely give them blankets, clothes, food and, most of all, His love for them. So, that's what I'm asking you in how you're applying what you're reading."

"I hear you, Preach, but I still won't ever trust the inmates in here, no matter what you say."

I told him I understood, but inside I knew a lesson was coming for Ray—soon.

All that week, Ray fought off the usual coffee beggars. His commissary bag was larger than any inmate's I'd seen before, and it brought swarms of inmates constantly begging. What did they have to lose? He was either going to say yes or no, and every time, his answer was an emphatic "No!" He wouldn't give in to any of them.

There was this one older black Jamaican inmate named Ponty. His hair was always pretty matted because he couldn't afford to keep it up. He had nobody on the outside, therefore he was forgotten. He'd probably hadn't enjoyed commissary in years. He'd always come around begging for coffee shots from those who'd gotten it. He'd say, with a big, gregarious smile on his face in a strong Jamaican accent, "Hey, my brother, can you give me, an island man who's been stuck in this place for many years, a shot of coffee?" Most of the time somebody would, but when he came up to Ray, who was now opening his huge bag and taking inventory, I thought Ray was going to jump off his bunk and kill him.

"Man, if you don't get yo' begging ass away from me, I'll come down there and strangle you!" he told him.

He scared Ponty so bad, he ran off. I told Ray that the Jamaican was harmless.

"See, that's how they come around and try to take advantage of you. But not me; I don't fall for it like you do."

Ray went into his bag and pulled out this huge jar of hair grease. I hadn't seen a jar of grease that big in years. When Ray opened it, Ponty came running back over. The poor guy probably hadn't had grease in his hair in years, maybe that's why he was willing to chance coming back to ask Ray for some of it.

"Hey, my brother, can a poor island man get a little bit of that for his tired hair?"

This time I begged Ray to let him have just a small bit for his hair. I was surprised when he reluctantly extended the jar out to him. Ponty scooped his hand into the jar, taking almost half of it. Even I was shocked at how much he'd taken. I just knew Ray would feel this proved his point.

"You crazy fool! See, Preach! Look how much he took! I ought to jump down from here and kill your ass! I tried being nice, but look what I get. See, I told you that crap doesn't work in here. I ain't never doing that again!"

By this point, Ponty was running through the dorm, probably thinking Ray was surely going to kill him now. I even felt it myself. He was truly incensed. But I said to him—even knowing he wouldn't understand in that moment, "God's telling me you should have given him the entire jar."

"What? He's lucky I don't break his damn neck for that! And now you're telling me that God's telling you I should have given him the entire jar? Preach, that one's gonna be a bit hard for me to believe He told you that."

I knew he didn't believe me, but in time I knew he would. It took a minute for Ray to cool down on that one. I felt bad for him. Every few minutes, he kept bringing it back up. I understood how he felt. Nobody wants to feel used, but I just knew there was a message coming for Ray.

After a while, the dorm finally went back to normal, and it was time for my Bible study with the inmates. They all came around with their Bibles, and we got started. I asked Ray to join us, but I could tell he was still pissed. I somehow didn't blame him, but I knew a lesson was coming for me to show him. That's when I asked him to jump down from his bunk. I wanted to show him something God was giving me in that moment for him to learn. Still thinking I was crazy, he slowly climbed down from his bunk and joined the circle of inmates.

"Watch Ray!" I told him as I put my arm on his shoulder. "It's all starting to happen for you now. Do you know why earlier I asked you to bless Ponty, the Jamaican inmate, and give him the entire jar of hair grease?"

He said no with a surprised look on his face. He then reminded me of how he'd tried to be nice to him, but he'd tried to scoop out all of it.

"Ray, Ponty one day told me he hasn't gotten a blessing in here for some time now. God was trying to use you to give him that blessing. Here's why. Because you can't take it with you—watch! That's when I cupped my hand to my right ear, and at that exact moment, over the loudspeaker came the sheriff's command, "Ray Morgan! Roll it up for release!"

"No way! How did you know that? They never tell us when we're getting shipped out! That was incredible! Oh my God!"

"Ray, the reason you should have given him the entire jar is because when you walk over to that door in a few minutes to leave, they're going to go through all of your items and throw most of it away, including that jar of grease you should have blessed Ponty with."

He was still in shock!

"Ray, now you're beginning to see how subtle God's message for us can be sometimes."

At that minute, the entire group, including me, surrounded Ray and just stood there and gave him a hug. In all of his days going in and out of jail, he was feeling genuine spiritual love from other inmates. He was still in shock, but in that moment he just stood there and tried to take it all in the best he could, not thinking that everyone was out to get him. Tears streamed down his face. It was such a beautiful thing to witness. When he'd first come to the jail dorm he'd had a calloused heart and wanted to beat up everyone in it. He reached down inside his bag, pulled out the remainder of the grease, and handed it to me.

"Preach, do me a favor. Please bless him with this for me."

"I would be honored, my brother."

"Ray Morgan! We said roll it up for release!"

Ray grabbed his large duffel bags and ran for the door. He stopped and ran back to give me his information on the outside. He said it was his sister's cell and I could always reach him through her. When I walked over and surprised Ponty with the jar, he broke down. Then he thanked me.

I pointed my finger in the air and said in a Jamaican accent, "I'm just the messenger, my brother!"

Ponty laughed, commenting on how bad my accent was. Just witnessing how something so little had meant so much to someone.

One day, they rushed in, put Ponty on a stretcher, and took him away. We never saw him again after that day. I later overheard from another inmate who knew him well that he'd died from cancer. That really saddened me. It just wasn't the same around the jail dorm after Ponty died. I would miss his jovial laugh and accent throughout the dorm every commissary day as he made his rounds begging for coffee shots.

Since then, I've always wanted to see Ray again so I could tell him that despite his worries about being taken advantage of, he had blessed a man and given him some happiness for a minute in his life. And he'd done it all with a simple jar of hair grease.

THE IRONY IN A SIGN

I was into about the third hour of my meditation one day when I received a vision again, showing me telling Steve months previously that his mother was going to die. It was unfortunate that she did die later that week. I tried to do all I could to help him get through it, to help assuage his pain.

There was also a vision telling me there would be one for myself as well. I was now feeling something, that May 3—the date when I'd tried to commit suicide in 2013—would somehow attach itself to my mother. I wasn't given any more than that. It was troubling, to say the least. I finished my meditation for the day, but the thought stayed with me for the rest of it. Little did I know it would reveal itself sooner than I'd thought.

The last time I saw my mother was May 3, 2014. She passed on May 4, 2014.

THE DEAL

The date was March 11, 2014. I knew this day would be special, especially after what China, my daughter, had told me.

I'd now lost track of how many times I had appeared in front of the judge. It had become routine. I had to get up and prepare myself before leaving to go. I was mentally and physically worn out, but I had to keep fighting my case. There was no way I was going to accept a sentence I didn't deserve. I couldn't help thinking about the vision I'd had the day before about my mother. The last time I'd spoken to her she'd seemed fine. I was hoping this one wasn't real. That would be too much to bear. I also thought about the spiritual work I had done with the inmates. I was still dedicated. Would I be deserting them if I left? I was now torn between the two.

Within a few minutes I heard the call over the loudspeaker to line up for the court line. I got dressed and headed out. I was expecting another usual day in court—a stalemate. The bus dropped us off about 7.30 a.m. The sheriff checked us in, then escorted some of us to the black inmate waiting tank. As I waited to see my attorney, I thought about my incarceration. What a ride it had been! It was nothing short of surreal. I hoped I'd saved some souls. The real test would come when they were released. Would they stay with the program and not come back to that living hell ever again?

I was finally escorted to the attorneys' floor. Half-an-hour passed until mine finally arrived. Judging by his smile he looked like he had good news. He said he'd received several character letters from friends. I told him that was great and how appreciative I was, and to thank them for me. He said he would. Then he said I had a new judge.

Out of nowhere, he asked me, "Did you really write all those songs?" he

I told him yes.

"Once the prosecutor hears this, you'll definitely get released. That is a good thing."

I'd had such bad luck with judges during my time of being incarcerated that I pretty much had to see it for myself before I believed it. The way it normally worked was that your attorney goes in first to plead your case in front of the judge. The judge makes his or her decision, then the sheriff cuffs you (you are oblivious to what had been discussed) and walks you into the court.

The sheriff led me over to a seat near my attorney. He quickly briefed me on what had been said. While we sat waiting for the judge to come out of his chambers, my attorney went over to the prosecutor, who would usually turn and look at me as if I were a murderer. My attorney fiddled with his iPhone, and the next thing I knew, *Stickwitu*, the song I'd co-written for The Pussycat Dolls, was now blaring all over the courtroom. I couldn't believe it! The prosecutor looked over and asked if I had really written it. It was one of his daughter's favorite songs.

Then the judge entered. My attorney and the prosecutor approached the bench. I could see the prosecutor now had a big smile on his face. After a few minutes, the judge had me stand with my attorney. He said he was going to make me an offer I couldn't refuse, and it would be my only offer. He now had my full attention. He told me he had read my file, along with the character letters, and that all the other judges had wanted to give me a felony strike with three years of probation.

"Here's my one-time deal for you," he said. "You've been here way too long. If you're willing to show the court you can attend a weekly mental health program for a year-and-a-half, then come back to court every three months with a progress report proving it, I'm willing to reduce the felony strike to a misdemeanor and drop the three-year probation. You also can expunge it from your record in a year. Well, Mr. Palmer, what is your decision?"

My attorney kept nodding his head like he was bobbing for apples. He was that excited.

"Yes, Your Honor, I'll take the deal," I answered with trepidation.

"You're free to leave right now," the judge said.

I asked if I could make a request, and I asked if I could be released on the 18th of the month. He laughed and said he'd never seen a released inmate who wanted to stay longer. I had reasons that they wouldn't understand. I wanted to go back to the dorm to finish my spiritual work with the inmates. I didn't want them to think I had abandoned them like so many others they'd told me about. The judge gave me seven days before my release date.

I went back to County that day. The inmates gathered around me and asked if I was leaving or staying. I hated to break the news to them, but I told them my time had finally run out. It was time for me to leave. It was bittersweet. I told them the deal I had taken. They said it was an amazing deal. Some wanted me to stay, which meant a lot to their spirits, while others said it was time for me to get back to my family.

Earl and the rest of the guys came over to hug me and wish me well. Earl was facing life for murder. I asked him to "always include your victims and their families in your prayers at night. Even if you're never getting out of here, with God, your spirit can be free of this place, if you're willing to surrender it. Remember the work we've done. Show God you have remorse and pray for redemption, grace, and forgiveness."

I told them I had seven days to work with them. I was thankful to each inmate who had come to my Bible studies, and wished them well. I had been transferred to twelve dorms in my time there, and had lost track of how many inmates I'd had the pleasure of ministering to. It had to have been close to one thousand! I can truly say it had been extremely spiritually rewarding, beyond comprehension for the inmates and me. God is truly a Savior of lost souls, starting with my own.

THE COST OF FREEDOM

Those seven days before my release seemed to pass slowly at first. I tried spending most of it praying with quite a few inmates, sometimes all night, for as many who needed it. They knew I was leaving, so quite a few requested it. I'd seen firsthand how men, myself included, responded to being in hell. Incarceration can break a man's spirit like a bronco rider on a wild horse in just a matter of time, especially if he has no spiritual foundation. Without it he could wind up lost and caught up in the gang politics within the system, beat somebody down, and have charges added to his sentence.

Being not so torn about leaving, would have made things much easier for me. I wished I had a few more months to pray and work with them. I just wanted to reach one more person. I would hate to see them let it go to the wayside once they were released. I was very passionate about the work I'd done up to that point. As I waited for the guard to call my name, I reflected on my time served. I couldn't help but remember that day on April 18, 1985, when I'd died. I know I went somewhere. I know I got a glimpse of heaven; I'm sure of it. That's where these visions had to come from.

I'd learned so much from being incarcerated. When I walked in there almost a year ago, I'd wanted to kill myself. I was suffering from depression. I had chronic joint pain, which still miraculously hadn't returned, praise God. And my relationship with Him was now amazing. It was truly a gift that showed me there was no limit to what the human spirit can do once we surrendered it to Him. I was determined that whatever was happening around me would not get the best of me. I practiced being *in* it, not *of* it. It was like having a spiritual shield of armor, which in time, made me immune to the violence and politics around me. That was where heavy prayer and seven hours a day of meditation for almost a year had made a difference. My spirit was somewhere soaring in a cloud, and I wanted to show other inmates how to let theirs reach those same heights.

Jail is a place where dreams come to die and are buried alive right in front of you. To make matters worse, I believe most people incarcerated in the L.A. County Jail would agree that the squalid conditions were deplorable. Rats and roaches everywhere. Rusted bunks and worn-out mattresses. As an inmate, it wasn't long before I discovered the isolating effect it had on me at first. Even when I was around other inmates, I was still in a world of my own. You have to be cautious at all times of your surroundings, unless you're in solitary, where, if you stayed long enough, you could lose your mind like so many had. Depending on the level you were classified, you had to be on high alert, especially if it was a level seven or eight, where I frequently ended up. A race riot could break out at any minute. Or you could piss off a lifer who had nothing to lose.

I found the conditions in the Yellows (psychiatric ward) to be neglectful. There were a lot of inmates with serious mental health problems who simply didn't belong in jail. (L.A. County Jail has the largest mental facility in the country.) Most of the inmates there should have been transferred to a mental hospital environment. They were being overlooked because of staff shortages and an outright lack of care management. They subsequently roamed around the dorms doing strange and disturbing things that are too graphic to write about. Or, there was the possibility one of them shanking and killing you in your sleep, yet not even realizing what he'd done. Could he rightfully be blamed if he was mentally incapacitated? He would more than likely wind up in Patton State Hospital for the criminally insane.

The thing I found fascinating was that some inmates knew the Bible inside out, like the back of their hands, yet they were illiterate. They could passionately quote you any Scripture from it but, in that same breath, couldn't read a regular book. I wrote letters for a lot of them. The sad part about it was some didn't take advantage of the programs available to teach them how to read. On the other hand, a lot of them did, and changed their lives as a result.

Some inmates felt God had abandoned them. This was the reason so many had lost their faith. These were the hardest to reach spiritually. In time, I befriended quite a few of them, but it took a lot of grueling work. That was why I felt so sad about the timing of my leaving—just when I was getting some of the tougher inmates to believe in God again. For some, it was their first time.

I saw firsthand the need for more spiritual counseling in jail that came from the older inmates working directly with the younger gang members. Those who were lifers or who had long sentences could really do some great work with them. The chaplains were doing a great job, but the only problem for some (not all) was that as soon as some of the gang members went back to their dorm/cell, they were right back to fighting again—therefore forgetting what just had been learned. I found that working with them every day produced unbelievable changes. It seemed impossible, but I witnessed it firsthand.

There are also men in there who want to change their lives, but just don't know how. I soon learned it wasn't just the words that were spoken that brought them to tears. It was also the compassion given to the little boy inside them who had been hiding all that time behind an adult with a calloused and broken soul.

Some of the inmates told me they were being heard for the first time on a spiritual level. I tried to be sincere when I listened to their problems. Sometimes hearing about their tough childhoods could be very disturbing and revealing but, most of all, sad. We'd sit there for hours and pray into the night, then they'd walk over to their bunk and sleep like a kitten. One inmate told me he hadn't slept with both eyes closed in jail for over thirty years.

Some, in the end, would have a breakthrough. They were grateful for that. Most of the time, they just wanted to know if God was truly merciful and forgiving, and had heard their pleas about the hard life they'd lived. I always tried to lead them to salvation and repentance. Sometimes that was challenging and/or virtually impossible to get across to some, especially the agnostics and atheists. Despite it, I still wasn't willing to give up on them.

It made me speechless witnessing some of their amazing transformations. I became passionate when I spoke to any of them, regardless of ethnic background. My heart truly felt for those who wanted to change their lives. In jail, you can't fake it. For the inmates who are spiritual, they can see right through you if you aren't sincere. Most of the time I had to be careful and choose my words accordingly. I had to earn their respect before talking to them about God; I learned that early on. God was the one thing some inmates revered and respected above all else. They took Him very seriously. It was truly an experience for me. I feel a lifetime's worth of self-healing happened in that place. Who would've thought you could find heaven while sitting in the middle of hell?

The time for me to leave had now finally come, sooner than I had anticipated. Here, I had gone the distance from being on suicide watch to a spiritual prayer counselor to inmates. That was the power of the Holy Spirit living and shining brightly within me. You never knew how He was going to use you once you surrendered to Him.

With minutes left, I began to wonder how I would integrate back into society. I still wanted to continue God's work on the outside. Go out and feed the homeless maybe? A deeper passion for them had developed in me in the past year after what I'd survived. God had used me in a way to bring spiritual change for so many locked behind iron bars.

"Palmer! Line it up for release!"

Finally, my last time hearing a sheriff's command. The echoes of it were still reverberating in my head when the bus pulled in to take me to court for my release.

The old cell door was cranked open as I gathered together my few belongings. As I passed other inmates in their cells, they wished me luck on the outside. Some yelled out, "Preach, don't forget us!"

Without any words spoken, I just nodded back, as I now understood the cost of freedoms: freedom from pain. Freedom from suicide. And now, freedom from jail. I now cherished and praised the God who had released me from them all and given me back my life.

PART 3

THE MORNING DISRUPTION

On the morning of October 30, 2018 I was awakened from a deep slumber by the distinct chime of my iPad notifying me I had email messages. I'd now been out of the L.A. County Jail for four years and was renting a room from an old friend. It was the usual early-morning hour of promotional emails, piling up and vying for my attention, offering unheard-of deals before my day had barely gotten started.

I was expecting mail from a potential client, and just as I turned over to go back to sleep I opened my iPad to check my messages. What I discovered in those next few moments would alter someone else's life hundreds of miles away in Portland, Oregon, and mine in Arizona forever from that day forward.

It was a link to one of the more popular genealogy sites, notifying me of a DNA match. I had been receiving them for years, ever since I'd had mine done. I had responded to hundreds of links that were mainly matches of first through eighth cousins—mostly distant. But this particular email was different: it said Parent/Child. There was a generic pale-blue illustration of a male and the name Kary Youman below it. This was all I had to go on. I was sure, on his end, that all he saw was the same picture, only with the name Robert D. Palmer below it.

I knew this had to be a mistake. Possibly a misprint. Maybe they'd confused my DNA with someone else's? Yet, I knew none of these possibilities were true. The matches were always accurate, especially when the probability rate was "extreme." My thoughts were now racing out of control.

All the time I was wondering, *'Who could this person possibly be? Who is his mother? How old is he? Who does this person already believe his father is? Would this disrupt his entire family?'*

These were just some of the mounting questions to consider, and it seemed as if the world in my room suddenly stopped in wait of a decision: whether to hit the link to the genealogy site, or to simply ignore it for now. That answer seemed to be stuck between floors, somewhere in the elevator of building anxiety, as I impatiently waited, thinking, *'This, and I haven't even had my morning coffee yet!'* I could only imagine what lay in store for the rest of that day.

As if it developed a mind of its own, my finger hit the link to the site, taking me directly to the DNA match. I stared in disbelief at the amount of DNA segments we shared; more than my brother and sister combined! The results were now indisputable. With eyes focused on the small green box with the bold word *Message* in it, I wondered, *'What do I do next?'*

The Messages

10:20 A.M.

I needed a moment to take it all in, so I poured my morning roast, took a mental step back, and breathed. The coffee was a little hotter than I normally liked, so I put it down to cool, then pulled up Miles Davis on my playlist. I needed to hear some music to calm me before deciding what to write in the message to this stranger named Kary Youman. I turned it up just loud enough to drown out the doubt swirling through my thoughts. *Milestones* was always a great song for that. Miles's trumpet was reminiscent of a Baptist minister preaching a sermon, and Lord knew I needed one that day. I wanted to be ready to face years of questions this young man might have for me. Would I be able to answer any of them?

2:00 P.M.

It took a few hours to think about it all. I lay my head on my pillow and proceeded to write him this message:

"Dear, Kary. Hi, my name is Robert Palmer. I checked my DNA matches today and I ran across yours. I'm actually in extreme shock at this minute! It says that you are definitely my son. I checked your DNA matches against my immediate family, and yours lines up with every single one of theirs. Absolutely

amazing! I would love to know more about you. My curiosity is peaking here!"

What seemed like days were only a few minutes before a return message popped up on my screen! The son, whose DNA only hours ago had just matched mine, responded:

"I'm just as shocked as you are, and this has always been a touchy subject for me."

He then asked if I knew his mother. He told me her name, but it didn't prick my memory; it just seemed too long ago. I wanted to be careful and not sound insulting, so I asked him how old he was, hoping it would give me a better timeframe of who she could be. He said he was thirty-six and would be thirty-seven that coming November, which meant he had been born in '81.

"Where were you in 1981?" he asked.

I responded that I was living in L.A. at that time. This would have put me somewhere in my late twenties. I asked him if he had some pics of his mom and himself, then and now. "I would love to see what you both look like."

I rummaged through some pictures to send him as well. Soon a barrage of pictures of him and his mother appeared in my inbox He was a handsome young man, and I could immediately see the striking resemblance between his mother and myself. She was a good-looking woman, and yet, I still didn't recognize her. I wasn't sure how to say that in my next message. I was sure, if I were in his shoes, that I would wonder why a man whose DNA stated he was my father couldn't remember who my mother was. I was at a loss for words and wasn't sure where to go from there, hoping I wasn't being disrespectful in any way.

The message exchange went on for a while longer with more questions from Kary and with as many answers as I could provide him. Then, there was a long pause.

Just when I thought he'd given up on asking me anything else, or maybe this was some sordid prank, a phone number appeared on the screen.

THE CALL

By the second unanswered ring, I found myself calming my shaking hand again as I took another sip of coffee.

'Sixty-five years old and my life is about to enter a whole new chapter.'

By the third ring, there was finally an answer. The voice on the other end responded simply with, "Robert? Hi. It's really nice to finally meet you."

"Same here," I replied.

The first thing I instantly noticed in just those few words was the articulate tone of his voice. It was pleasant.

"I'm not quite sure where to start here. It says you're definitely my biological father. Obviously, you can only imagine how numb I must be at this moment and all the questions I have for you. There's just so much to know and to talk about with you. I hope you don't mind."

"No, I totally understand, Kary. It hasn't quite hit me yet either. It all still seems a bit surreal after waking up just a few hours ago to an email telling me about a son out of nowhere. I've been in a daze ever since! If I may ask, who did you grow up believing your biological father was?"

"Well, Robert, his name is George. To this day, we've never developed the type of bond I'd hope to have with my father. I love him dearly, I just wish our relationship was stronger. He and my mom unfortunately separated when I was young. One day the doctors told them that he wasn't my dad because he didn't have the sickle cell trait. I didn't find out about this until I was twelve, when my mom came into my room and shared the news with me. I felt like I'd been hit in the gut by Mike Tyson. It was that devastating!"

"Wow! I can't even imagine what that could have felt like, especially being so young. Do you and he still talk?"

"Rarely. Like I said, I wish it was better. I'm very close with his family. They've always been supportive and there for me throughout my life. They will always be family to me and that will never change, even though I've now found you, my biological father.

"Robert, you know I only recently did my DNA test, and for it to come back with these results so soon is still a bit hard to believe. I just can't say enough how this is all pretty amazing and a lot to take in at one time! I immediately called my mom after a few messages from you. I wanted to know if she knew who you were. I don't think she's gotten beyond the initial shock to even answer the question! I told her I didn't want to keep you waiting, and I'd call her back after I spoke to you. That's what took so long when you didn't hear back from me after a few minutes."

"I kinda figured that's what might've happened."

We talked about my other kids, his half-siblings, where they lived, what they were like, how old they were, and how many kids they had.

"So, after me sending you the pictures and you having some time to think about it all, do you now remember how you guys met?"

"You know what, Kary, I think maybe at this point I should give your mom a call and talk to her about that subject first, just out of respect, if you don't mind. I'll call you back and share with you after we've talked. It's really nice to be able to meet you. You really sound like a fine young man, just from this short conversation. Sounds like she did a great job in raising you; it says a lot about her. I'm hoping we can develop a relationship, if you're willing."

"I would like that. It's nice to finally meet you as well. And I agree, you're right. Here's her number. I know she can't wait to talk to you! I'm sure there's a lot for you guys to talk about. Oh, and, Robert, I have one last question, if you don't mind?"

"Sure, what's that?"

"I'm curious to know, do you have the sickle cell trait?"

"Yes, I do."

I also told him that most of my other kids had it as well. He sounded reluctant to believe it at first, which I understood. Maybe he thought it was a convenient answer at this point. I assured him I'd prove it when I called him back.

"Thanks, I'd appreciate it," he said with a sigh of relief.

After the call, I just stood there for a few minutes. No lingering afterthoughts, just a mind full of unexplainable silence. That's when I made the call to the mother of my son.

THE TRAIT

So far, the day was turning into an emotional whirlwind, a continuous unfolding of revelations and events. I'd decided that before calling Kary's mom I wanted to take a minute and go back to the year 1981. Maybe try to remember the timeline. Try to put together the missing pieces of how we'd met.

Within a few hours, it started to come back to me. It was now clearer. I had met Linda that February at a music industry party. I believe the reason we'd lost touch so quickly was because I'd just been hired at the last minute by the R&B group LTD to go on tour with them to Europe. Everything became a blur after that. We immediately went into extensive rehearsals for a few weeks, and I'd had to quickly get rid of my apartment and have my phone turned off.

In those days, there were no answering machines or cellphones. I'd put all my belongings into storage, and I was sure her number was somewhere in there. By the time I'd come back to the states months later, my life had changed, and I was sure hers had as well. More than likely, we'd just moved on with our lives—unfortunately, neither of us knowing that Kary was my son.

As far as the sickle cell trait was concerned, I'd totally forgotten about it years ago. It was shortly after confirming with my other kids that it was primarily an African American disease and they had it. After their moms and I educated them on how to deal with the disorder, it was then put to bed. Now that this young man had graced the fold of my offspring and the irony for a reason of its proof, I would be more than honored to provide the information if necessary. Especially, if in this case that was what it took, for the addition of traditional medical science to take precedence over the current medical advancements of DNA. After so many years, I knew they wanted closure. I was certain it still rested heavily on the two of them, and I was now prepared to do whatever it took to prove it.

When Linda (Kary's mother) answered the phone, I could hear the jovial laughter of a child in the background.

"Robert? Oh, hold on a minute, let me quiet my grandson."

"What's his name?"

"His name is Darius."

"What a blessing to have grandkids. I have six myself. So, Linda, it's my pleasure to be able to finally talk to you after all these years. How are you after hearing this news only a few hours ago?"

"Robert, after all these years, it's my pleasure to talk to you again as well. Deep down in my heart, I'm so happy for the both of you. It's truly been a lot of years of wanting to have closure to this. I hope you can see beyond my skepticism at this point. You have to understand, it was so many years ago."

She went on to tell me how she'd just started dating a man named George, whom she'd thought was

Kary's dad around that time. The timelines were so close and our meeting each other had been so brief, she'd just assumed he was the father. I told her I understood, and I had taken a minute before calling to try to put together the timeline of events; how we'd met and what could've happened afterwards. After sharing it with her, she agreed it made a lot of sense, but her reservations were still there because of the sickle cell part. It wasn't that she mistrusted the science of DNA, she just needed closure about the doctor's sickle cell finding years ago. It was all she'd had to go on at that time, and for her, the biological father had to have the trait.

"So, Robert, do you have the trait?"

"Yes, I do have it, Linda."

"Can you show me the proof that you do?"

I asked her to hold the line while I looked through my medical records. I must have scoured through boxes and boxes of files. I just knew it had to be there, but I wasn't having any luck. I pulled out more boxes and went through those, but still no luck. I could feel the tension mounting and her growing impatience.

PROOF

Unfortunately, I was down to the last box. At that point, I didn't know what to tell her. I felt I'd let her down. I knew she needed the proof; it wasn't personal. As I went back to the phone to tell her, I remembered I'd gone to a new doctor a few months back. He'd asked for my medical records and those records were in the drawer. I ran over to it and pulled it so hard that all the files fell to the floor! Like a mad man, I was scurrying around on my knees, searching through the pile. Finally, there it was! Clear as day! All the way down at the bottom of the document, it said: Sickle cell anemia trait.

"Linda, here it is! I found it!" I yelled out in relief.

"Oh my God, Robert! Lord knows how long I've waited for this moment. It has to be over twenty-something years. Can you take a picture of it and send it to me now?"

After taking the picture, I looked at my iPhone, and when it said 'Delivered' a few seconds later, that soft-spoken voice on the other end of the line was now crying joyous tears.

THE CONVERSATIONS

After talking to Kary's mom and showing her the lab work that confirmed the sickle cell trait, I called my son back. I knew he would have a thousand questions for me. And he did! That first day alone, we talked for over six hours. Our first conversations were mostly about getting acquainted with one another. We exchanged quite a few pictures between us, laughing at the similarities and moving close to tears when we shared some of the more in-depth stories.

These conversations went on for months. Later my son was invited to speak at TEDx Portland and share how we'd met online through a DNA service. I knew TEDx was a high-profile event. I was proud of him for having the courage to share our story, and impressed by the grace he showed on stage. A few months after his talk, he invited me to visit him in Portland to meet face-to-face and do an interview with the local news station, which was now interested in hearing more of our story.

I'd had a forty-plus-year career in the music industry, so I was used to being on television, but it had been so long since I'd done anything in front of a camera that I was reluctant. I hadn't worked out in almost two years and needed to get some dental work done. His openness and kind heart truly touched me. I was inspired to get my life back together, so I joined a gym and scheduled time with my dentist.

A few months passed before I landed in Portland to visit my son and immediately fell in love with the place. The vibrant neighborhoods, mild weather, and abundance of trees were enough for me. Kary and I got along very well, and I enjoyed spending time with him and meeting some of his close friends. After being there for only a week, I knew I wanted to spend the rest of my life there.

DON'T DISTURB THE GROOVE

Once I arrived back in Arizona, I knew my days there were numbered. I'd been depressed for almost a year and couldn't stand my living situation. Several months after visiting Portland, Kary and I arranged for him to fly down to Arizona to help me pack and move. We planned to load my belongings in a U-Haul and hitch it to my car so we could drive up to Portland, where I'd now committed to becoming a resident. I was grateful because Kary had introduced me to a good friend of his named Gene who had a room available for rent. I'd never met the guy but I trusted my son, so I was excited to have a place to call home. The GPS said it would take us about fifteen hours to drive from Las Vegas to Portland, straight through.

The ride is one I'll never forget because we had a chance to bond through the power of music. We sang, laughed, and spoke about a range of artists, from Jimmy Page to Jimi Hendrix. We talked about politics and debated our favorite films. Time flew by, and before we knew it we were pulling into Portland. Kary offered to drive several times during the trip, but I was in the zone. I didn't want to offend him, but I wasn't tired and I enjoyed driving these days as much as I loved music.

In total, I drove seventeen-and-a-half hours. I think my excitement and obsessive personality gave me the strength to push through and keep going in spite of the cramp I was starting to feel in my lower back. It was the first time in over a year I felt at peace. This was the beginning of a new chapter. ***Praise God!***

Epilogue
by Kary Youman

After thirty-seven years of not knowing each other, it was surreal to now have my biological father living in the same state as me. He would always tell me that his greatest hope was to one day have all of his kids (six of us) in one place, united and working together as a family. Shortly after moving to Portland, my youngest sister and brother relocated from Hawaii and Florida, respectively, to be closer to our dad. I could see a glimpse of hope in his eyes the first time we all met up to spend time together in person. I'll never forget that moment.

My dad was passionate about giving back. He wanted to create a music charter school for underserved communities in the Portland Metro Area, and I remember staying up late with him many nights over the phone, discussing the ins and outs of bringing his vision to life. By then, I knew this project would be a lot to handle mentally, so I tried to take on as much as I could to support him. I encouraged him to reach out to some of his friends in the music industry to see if they wanted to partner with us in helping lay the curriculum's foundation. I built a website for the academy and connected my dad with friends who were passionate about the craft.

There was some momentum early on, but Dad's focus shifted elsewhere after a few mental setbacks. To combat this tendency, I suggested we focus on one project at a time. From our first conversation over the phone, we had talked about writing books, but we didn't consider working on one together until we met in person for the first time in June 2019. I knew, if we couldn't raise the funds and attract the right team to launch the charter school right away, we could at least make time to work on a book together.

Collaborating with Dad was an intense experience. Initially, we couldn't agree on the best way to approach our story. We went back and forth about the title, book cover design, and a format that would make the most sense. One night, he and I hung up from a conversation that felt like days. The following morning, he sent me a voice memo saying he'd been up all night writing. In five hours, he had typed more than forty thousand words. I couldn't register how that was even possible. In hindsight, it's clear that my father was on the creative side of mania that evening. What initially had started as a book about the conversations he and I had during our first year getting to know each other morphed into his life story and how he'd gone *From Misery to Hope*.

A week has passed since my sister called on New Year's Eve to tell me Dad was no longer with us. I still have a hard time processing that I will never speak with him again on this plane of reality. He and I talked at least once a week on the phone, but we would text and leave voice memos several times throughout the day to check in with each other. The last time I heard his voice was four days before he took his life. He hadn't slept in his bed for two weeks.

I later found out he had stopped taking his medications and had vowed never to go back to the hospital for treatment because he was tired of being treated like a guinea pig. After several rounds of Electroconvulsive Therapy (ECT) and being prescribed many different medications to regulate his depression, Dad had no lasting relief from the pain and the sorrow he experienced in his mind. I think he had finally given up on treatment and the mental health system altogether.

I will never know what the last few moments of Dad's life were like, but I know the love I have for him and the bond we created will never die. The number of people who struggle with some form of mental illness is alarming. Since his passing, my family and I have committed to honoring Dad's legacy by sharing his story and becoming advocates for mental health awareness.

If you or someone close to you has been diagnosed with a mental disorder and is struggling to get by, please seek help. We have listed a few resources in the Appendix. There are dozens of organizations nationwide that can help and support you and your loved ones on this journey. You are not alone.

AFTERWORD
(EXCERPTED FROM ROBERT'S CELEBRATION OF LIFE EULOGY)
BY GLORIA PALMER

Robert was a son, a brother, a father, a grandfather, an uncle and cousin, a friend and a colleague to many. Robert started out in the ninth grade playing the drums. Then he and two of his friends decided they were going to start a band. One friend said he was going to play the bass guitar and Robert said he was going to play drums, but his other friend bullied Robert into letting him play the drums, so Robert chose guitar also.

Robert received his first guitar at the age of 13, and it was on and poppin' after that. He was self-taught, practicing sometimes seven days a week for up to fourteen hours a day. The name of his first official band was The Booty People, and he got his first big break in the 1970's when his band was signed by the Los Angeles-based, legendary group, WAR. He made up his mind he was going to be somebody in the music world and made numerous sacrifices, eventually achieving Grammy-nominated success in 2006. Ironically, his Grammy nomination was not for his extraordinary talent as a guitarist. It was for songwriting.

Robert was an accomplished guitarist, record producer, Grammy-nominated songwriter, a mentor, consultant, touring musical director, and he scored films. He felt he had been so blessed in his extensive music career to have had over forty years of contributions, covering various areas of the music industry. Robert has entertained multitudes all over the world with the mastery of his guitar. Over his career he had the privilege of working with Prince, Chaka Kahn, The Pussycat Dolls, Avant, Lionel Richie, Deniece Williams, Natalie Cole, Billy Preston, The Gap Band, Miles Davis, Smokey Robinson, Will Downing and Little Richard, just to name a few.

When he moved from performance to song writing, he also felt he was blessed to learn from some of the best: Steve Kipner, Lindy Robbins, Ryan Tepper, Kasia Livingston, Siedah Garret, Franne Golde, Bonnie McKee, Brenda Russell, Leon Ware, and Judd Friedman. It was with Franne Golde and Kasia Livingston that he co-wrote the Grammy-nominated StikWitU, the song that was playing as you came into the Memorial Service.

But Robert was also a deeply troubled man. He suffered from bipolar depression. He would put on his mask to hide his pain, go out on stage and put on a stellar performance, then go back to his hotel room and medicate himself with drugs to dull the pain. No one knew. He was worried about how he would be perceived and received in the music industry if anyone knew. So he hid his pain for years, until he could hide it no longer. He went to therapists and took the prescription meds, to only get short-term relief.

On April 18th, 1985, Robert died of a heart attack. Dying was a peace Robert never knew existed, but just as quickly as he had been ripped from this world, he was jerked back—TWICE! From that moment on, Robert knew something had drastically changed inside of him. He didn't see the world the same, feeling that he now existed in a space between life and death. After his near-death experience, he developed an ever-increasing case of social phobia. Although his career in the music industry as a writer/producer continued to flourish, his life became unbearable.

Robert and I reconnected on a personal level in 2008 and became best friends. We would literally talk EVERY DAY, whether it was 5 minutes or 10 hours plus. Robert had such an incredible memory for facts and trivia, and there were many times when he blew me away with his depth of knowledge on so many different subjects. It would be 5/6 a.m., and Robert and I would be laughing like banshees over some funny story he was sharing, reminiscing about this or that, or something that had caught our attention in the news. There were many mornings when the sun came up on our conversations.

It was during this time that I learned of his mental illness, and sometimes we just talked about the depths of his pain. I had to learn to recognize the signs when his illness was in control and not be offended. When he was in the darkest places, Robert could be harsh, overbearing, relentless. We laughed, we argued, we forgave. Robert was amazing. He was talented, creative, intellectual, an interior designer (he could hook up your house or apartment), a chef, trivia and movie buff, he was meticulous and a perfectionist. I can't remember a year when Robert didn't predict the correct winner of Best Picture for the Oscars. Robert seemed to be so full of life that at times it was hard for me to correlate the depths of his pain with the heights of his joy, how someone who could make you laugh until tears were running down your face could also make the tears run down your face just hearing the sadness in his voice. But that's the nature of bipolar depression, what used to be known as manic-depressive disorder.

Robert's first attempt to end his life was in 2013, due to a psychotic break which caused an incident for which he ended up in L.A. County Jail for a year. The family was so concerned because Robert had never been locked up for any reason. But to our surprise, Robert actually found purpose in jail. Because we were raised in a Christian home, Robert knew of God, so he got back to building his relationship with God and God used him mightily. He told me of so many miracles that happened while he was there. I even have copies of some of the letters written by inmates to Robert about how God had used him to change their lives. He was respectfully referred to as Preach by inmates of all colors and nationalities.

I would like to read one of the letters he received. (Read letter from inmate.) That was the kind of impact Robert had on the inmates by allowing God to use him in a place that's considered a hellhole.

When he left L.A. County, he started his own program of feeding the homeless in Los Angeles. Wherever he saw them—at the park, on the corner, in alleys, by the freeway—he was moved with compassion to offer a cup of coffee, a meal, or money, and a kind word. Robert's primary message to the homeless was God loves you and He wants you to know He hasn't forgotten you. Eventually, with the help of a friend who donated food from a restaurant, he would go out every night and take food to the homeless. While living in Jacksonville, FL, he also volunteered with the Red Cross to help people who had been displaced from Hurricane Irma in Tampa in 2017.

After Robert's second attempt on his life in 2019, he decided to do Electroconvulsive Therapy (ECT). The oppression and darkness were overwhelming. He said he had tried everything else and he was at the end of his rope. He was willing to go to this extreme for a chance at peace and true happiness. You see, Robert still had hopes and dreams. For a while, after the first series of ECT treatments, there seemed to be an improvement in his condition. After visiting with his son Kary in 2019, he decided to move to Portland, Oregon. He said the place was beautiful and he was looking forward to finally having the peace he had sought his whole life. He was so optimistic, and in early 2020 he moved to Portland. Eventually, two of his other children, Bianca and Rob Jr., also moved to Portland.

But, unfortunately, it was not to be. The darkness and oppression returned with a vengeance. Robert went through another series of ECT treatments, but this time there was no improvement in his condition. He felt like it was worse. He talked about how he just couldn't get his hopes up again. I tried to get him to come visit, to raise his faith that the Lord had a miracle with his name on it, but he no longer had even that mustard seed of faith. Robert wanted desperately to live, but he was so broken and the oppression and torment were too much. He said he couldn't go back to the hospital. It was more frustration than help, especially with the COVID protocols.

Two weeks before Robert ended his life, he called me up and said, "Hey Sis, I want you to make me a promise."

I said, "Okay."

He said, "If anything happens to me, promise me you won't let me be forgotten?"

"Robert," I asked, "how could we ever forget you?"

He said, "No, promise me."

I said, "Okay, I promise."

You see, because of the darkness and oppression that were eating away at Robert's soul—his mind, his will, his feelings, his emotions, his thoughts—he didn't realize his value. He didn't see himself as the kind, loving, compassionate person he was. He could not see himself as his family and friends saw him. All he could see was his mistakes and he judged himself harshly for them.

The last time I talked to my brother was on my birthday. He called me and said, "Hey Sis, just calling to say Happy Birthday and I love you." The next day, he was gone. We always think we'll have more time.

It's time to take off the masks. Mental illness is a dirty little secret in black culture. Every family has that one person everyone whispers about. As the old folks used to say, "They're just a little touched in the head. That one right there, he/she ain't all there." I'm hoping Robert's life will challenge some of you to show compassion to that family member. Or, maybe it's a friend, who on some days is a little "different". Robert was tormented because he felt he had alienated so many of his friends with his disorder. Don't let how Robert left this world define your memories of him. Remember him for the funny, kind, loving, sentimental, and compassionate soul he really was. If you have negative or painful memories of some of your encounters, don't just throw them out. Remember his suffering and resolve to be one who will reach out to someone else who is suffering. Mental illness is a very lonely disease and so many are suffering in silence.

There's a saying: Seek first to understand, then to be understood. Too many times we only see our side of the equation and don't try to see the other side. Try having a conversation, but don't listen simply to respond. Listen to really hear what the other person is saying. It can be enlightening. Sometimes people who are hurting don't know how to ask for help, or they're afraid to ask, or they're ashamed. Think about how frightening it must be to have your own mind turn against you, but you don't want people to judge you or to think you're 'Looney Tunes.' If you'll tune your ear and your heart in, you will hear the sadness and the pain. Be a safe place, without judgment, for them to vent, but urge them to get help. Mental illness will make you withdraw from family and friends into a very dark place because of the stigma that is still attached to it, but it is in that aloneness that the torment and oppression really get a stronghold. Several celebrities have come out and talked about their fight against mental illness, hoping to bring it more into the spotlight to help remove the stigma.

If you have family members or friends where there are unresolved issues, I urge you to try to resolve them. Everyone won't be amenable to resolving the issues, but at least your conscience will be clear that you tried. If someone has reached out to you but you turned that person away, think about it. Is there a way to resolve the issue? It's truly sad how many relationships have been torn apart over a misunderstanding. If you can, talk it out. Forgive those who have hurt you, whether they ask for it or not. Not only for their sakes, but for your own. Forgiveness is a beautiful thing. It gives people the grace to make mistakes and those mistakes not be held over their heads forever. The Word says, if we don't forgive, then we won't be forgiven by our Heavenly Father. If you are the one who has wronged someone else, ask for forgiveness then forgive yourself. Robert made it a point to reach out to many in this last year to ask for forgiveness, but Robert didn't know how to forgive himself for the things he felt he had done wrong.

I think of Robert's last moments here on earth, and sometimes, my grief, guilt, and sadness are too much to bear. Grief that he really is gone, guilt because I feel I didn't fight hard enough for him, and sadness that he felt so alone in his last days. So, I give it to the One who bore it all for me. The Word says, For God so loved the world that He gave His only begotten Son, that whosoever believeth on HIM should not perish but have everlasting life. I know I will see my brother again in eternity because I know Robert believed.

If you haven't made Jesus Christ, Yahushua Ha'Mashiach, your Lord and Savior, if you haven't accepted the free gift of salvation by grace through faith in the death, burial, and resurrection of Jesus Christ, the completed work of the Son of the Living God on Calvary, who paid the ultimate price so you and I could have eternal life, I invite you to do so today. Tomorrow is promised to no one.

Robert Donnell Palmer. Born: December 19, 1953. Finally found his peace: December 31, 2020. RIP, Brother Dear. Your soul is finally beside the still waters. We loved each other dearly, without a doubt. You were deeply loved by many and you deeply loved many. You will never be forgotten. To God be the glory! I love you.

NOTE TO THE READERS

Even though Robert did not get his victory on this side, there are many who do. Don't ever give up hope. Don't ever give up fighting for your peace. Find that listening ear, that person(s) who will stick with you and pray you through the trials and challenges it takes to get to mental stability. Join a support group. Find a therapist who actually listens to you, especially when you say your meds aren't working. Keep looking up, love yourself, and give yourself some grace.

Appendix
Mental Health Organizations

American Foundation for Suicide Prevention
   www.afsp.org

Black Emotional and Mental Health
   www.beam.community

Black Men Heal
   www.blackmenheal.org

Black Mental Health Alliance
   www.blackmentalhealth.com

Black Mental Wellness
   www.blackmentalwellness.com

Hope For The Day
   www.hftd.org

Mental Health in America
   www.mentalhealthamerica.org

National Alliance on Mental Illness (NAMI)
   www.nami.org
   1-800-950-6264
   Or in a crisis, text "NAMI" to 741741 for 24/7

NATIONAL INSTITUTE OF MENTAL HEALTH (NIMH)
www.nimh.nih.gov

NATIONAL SUICIDE PREVENTION LIFELINE
www.suicidepreventionlifeline.org
1-800-273-8255

THE UYENO FOUNDATION
www.uyenofoundation.org

Made in the USA
Monee, IL
24 June 2021

72015286R00173